Dr Rachel Carlton Abrams gained her degrees at Stanford, UC San Francisco and Berkeley. She lives in California with her family where she chairs a committee for the Academy of Integrative Health and Medicine and practises at Santa Cruz Integrative Medicine.

'Dr Rachel Abrams is amazingly caring and conscientious. I have benefited from her considerable conventional medical knowledge as well as from her skill with natural remedies. She has kept a careful eye over my welfare all the way from California and has maintained a friendly and professional relationship with my South African doctors who have welcomed her contributions happily. It is because they have not been intrusive. My South African medical team and I hold her in very high regard and hope her book is as successful as it deserves to be for the benefit of even more people.'

God bless you.'
DESMOND TUTU,
Archbishop Emeritus of Cape Town

'Dr Rachel Abrams has written the bible for any woman wanting to hear the wise voice of her own heart, mind, and body. You know those complaints women share with each other over lunch, like fatigue, anxiety, low libido . . . ? Dr Abrams gives practical, holistic and brilliant ways to alleviate each one. Best of all, she empowers women to trust themselves and lead in their own healing. I'm giving this book to my daughter and every friend I have.'
JULIE SCHWARTZ GOTTMAN, PhD,
Co-founder and President, *The Gottman Institute*

'Rachel Abrams is a truly exceptional physician, who has the breadth of interest and intellect to consider a patient's entire experience, not just limited pathologies. Where many health books focus on limited topics, *BodyWise* considers a huge range of factors that may affect our well-being. Like its author, it offers abundant hope, wisdom, and practical measures to address a vast range of issues. I wish I could make *BodyWise* required reading for anyone who wants to live a full, rich, active, and healthy life.'
MARTHA BECK, bestselling author,
life coach and columnist for O, *The Oprah magazine*

'*BodyWise* quickly gets to the root of what ails you, showing how you can heal yourself by tuning in to what your symptoms are telling you. This is truly an extraordinary guide for becoming your healthiest self with the right combination of knowledge, self-care, and sense of humour.'
SARA GOTTFRIED MD, *New York Times* bestselling author of
The Hormone Cure and *The Hormone Reset Diet*

'With all the health and diet books flooding the market and ratcheting up our stress responses with overwhelm, it can be challenging for health-conscious individuals to know how to care for the body temple. Enter Rachel Carlton Abrams's *BodyWise*. It's not just that Rachel is the best doctor I know. It's that she has shown me that when you educate yourself about the many potential tools for enlivening your vitality and then tune into the deep wisdom inherent in your body's inner compass in order to discern what is right for you, you become your own doctor in ways no book and no physician can match. Whether you sense that your medicine is a nutritional shift, new tools for moving your body, prescribing love and community as medicine for the soul, optimizing your sex life, or getting in touch with your life's purpose in order to optimize your health, this book will support your whole health journey as it also connects you with the body wisdom that can guide you to creating a life your body loves.'

LISSA RANKIN, MD, *New York Times* bestselling author
of *Mind Over Medicine*

'Dr Abrams offers practical steps to get you feeling better and more in touch with your body. Whether you have pain, are wondering about hormone replacement therapy or simply want to improve your health, *BodyWise* offers you a path to success.'

MIMI GUARNERI, MD FACC, President of the *Academy of Integrative Health and Medicine* and author of *The Heart Speaks*

'Dr Rachel Abrams is a lifelong expert on women's health, and her new book *BodyWise* is a revelation – a guide to achieving total health and well-being written with the authority of a world class physician and the warmth of a dear friend. Packed with specific treatment advice and a paradigm-shifting view of whole body health, this book will empower you to be the healthiest, and happiest, version of yourself.'

MARK HYMAN, MD, author of the *New York Times* bestseller, *Eat Fat Get Thin*; Director, *Cleveland Clinic Center for Functional Medicine*

'Chronic fatigue, chronic pain, chronic sleep problems, anxiety/depression, weight gain, and a decrease in sexual function are a common list of problems I see in my practice every day . . . and often, all in the same individual. Dr Rachel Carlton Abrams has taken her 20 years of clinical experience, her research/insights/intuition and intellect to bear, in producing this resourceful book for men and women who have one or more of these problems. Readers can gain advice on common sense practical approaches, plus be exposed to some of the most well-known natural medicine therapies to approach their health issues. Self-help resources such as *BodyWise* . . . can help to turn a life towards the positive.'

TORI HUDSON, N.D. Author, *Women's Encyclopedia of Natural Medicine*; Clinical Professor, National University of Natural Medicine, Bastyr University and SW College of Naturopathic Medicine; Medical Director, A Woman's Time

'There is a common language and wisdom available to every human being since the beginning of time, a great treasure, which we can find if we take time to listen for it. This is what Dr Rachel Abrams, MD, teaches to us in this remarkable book. It is the language of our bodies and the wisdom which it brings to our consciousness is truly the truth we can learn and trust. It is the physician within each of us and it is what does the real healing. A surgeon can repair a wound but the life force within us does the healing and this is who you will meet and learn from as you study this book and age into health.'

GLADYS TAYLOR MCGAREY, MD, MD[H], Co-founder *American Holistic Medical Association* and the 'Mother of Holistic Medicine'

'*BodyWise* represents the remembering of our hearts – the wisdom voice within each of us that helps us to reconnect with the natural world, our friends and family, our purpose in this lifetime, and the awareness of our own intelligence. Dr Rachel has connected with the simple wisdom by truly listening to what people have been sharing with her for years as a healer – the wisdom of knowing what is out of balance and the receptivity, based upon her compassionate presence, to support the return to balance, to vibrant living, and to optimal health. We are blessed to hear the evolutionary expression of Dr Rachel's voice as a true healer and as a consummate teacher.'

PATRICK HANNAWAY, MD, President, *Institute for Functional Medicine*

'Dr Rachel Carlton Abrams has created a wonderful combination of concepts and stories, all geared toward teaching you how to listen to your body, tap into your inner wisdom and find the happy healthy life you are looking for. As a leader in the field of Integrative Medicine, Dr Abrams brings insight, experience and humour to her writing. I highly recommend this book for anyone yearning to find your inner wise self, that voice within that is waiting to welcome you with open arms.'

MOLLY M. ROBERTS, MD, MS, ABIHM, Past President of the *American Holistic Medical Association*, Board member of the *Academy of Integrative Health*

'*BodyWise* is a profoundly compassionate book that will help you to understand the messages your body is continually sending you. If you want to become more fully alive and vibrantly healthy, if you want to create a life with more love and less pain, *BodyWise* will show you the way. It is a superb guide to lifelong healing.'

JOHN ROBBINS, Author and President of *The Food Revolution Network*

'If you are looking to create health and vitality in your life, this is a must-read book that integrates science with the transformative power of curiosity to access inner wisdom so you can heal and thrive from within.'

DANIEL FRIEDLAND, MD, Founding Chair, *Academy of Integrative Health & Medicine*; CEO, *SuperSmartHealth*; author, *Leading Well from Within*

'Rachel Abrams has created the most comprehensive guide I've ever seen for women's health. By brilliantly showing how to use the body as the most reliable diagnostic tool for healing, Dr Abrams is paving the way for practitioners and patients alike to integrate body intelligence into wellness. This is a book worth having by your nightstand for sure!'

STEVE SISGOLD, author of *Whole Body Intelligence*

Dr Rachel Carlton Abrams

BodyWise

Discovering Your Body's Intelligence for Lifelong Health and Healing

Your comprehensive guide to more sleep,
better energy and better health

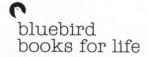

bluebird
books for life

First published 2016 by Rodale Books

First published in the UK 2017 by Bluebird
an imprint of Pan Macmillan
20 New Wharf Road, London N1 9RR
Associated companies throughout the world
www.panmacmillan.com

ISBN 978-1-5098-1650-7

This book is intended as a reference volume only, not as a medical manual.
The information given here is designed to help you make informed decisions
about your health. It is not intended as a substitute for any treatment that
may have been prescribed by your doctor. If you suspect that you have a
medical problem, we urge you to seek competent medical help.

Pan Macmillan does not have any control over, or any responsibility for,
any author or third party websites referred to in or on this book.

1 3 5 7 9 8 6 4 2

A CIP catalogue record for this book is available from the British Library.

Printed and bound by CPI Group (UK) Ltd, Croydon, CR0 4YY

Visit **www.panmacmillan.com** to read more about all our books
and to buy them. You will also find features, author interviews
and news of any author events, and you can sign up for e-newsletters
so that you're always first to hear about our new releases.

For Jesse, Kayla, and Eliana.
You heal my heart every day.

Contents

INTRODUCTION

The Key to Your Health and Well-Being Lies Inside You

have been a primary-care physician (similar to a general practitioner in the UK) for more than 2 decades on the front lines of modern medicine, hearing the health issues women struggle with most. I have held the hands and hearts of countless patients as they share the pain and suffering that these issues have caused in their lives. At least 75 per cent of my patients have the same constellation of complaints.

They're tired. They don't sleep well. They've lost their sex drives. They suffer from some kind of chronic pain, such as headaches, back pain, or pelvic pain. They experience depression, anxiety, or both. And quite often, they also have allergies, autoimmune problems, or some other sign of their bodies attacking themselves. They may not have all of these symptoms at once, but they often have most of them over time. I certainly have.

For years, I kept asking myself why so many women have some or all of these symptoms. Could this really just be coincidence? Might these symptoms all be connected? And might there be a way to address them together?

As an integrative (or holistic) physician, I am fortunate to have the time to really listen to my patients and to hear what is behind their symptoms. I schedule an entire hour with my new patients to hear about their concerns and complaints and learn about their lives in great detail. Over and over, women talk to me about the same life challenges. My patients feel pulled in multiple directions by their many roles and responsibilities. They feel torn between taking care of their families and friends and performing at work. They are overwhelmed and exhausted by the blessing and burden of all their commitments. They answer society's call to be 'superwomen,' yet regardless of the age and life stage, from recent college graduates in their twenties to retirees in their seventies, so many women are depleted by their lives. They are quite perceptive about their busy worlds, but they

> Listening to your body is not just about avoiding future illness. It is about wellness and vitality now and about your being able to have the life you – and your body – will love.

lack deep intelligence about their most important instrument – their bodies. My general practice colleagues see a similar epidemic of these symptoms. This set of complaints is so common that I have come to see it not just as a random collection of symptoms but instead as its own diagnosis: chronic body depletion.

Chronic body depletion occurs because of the demands that modern life puts on our bodies and because we have lost touch with our bodies' intelligence. Many women in my practice and among my friends and family have come to accept extraordinary levels of pain and discomfort as normal, not realizing that their bodies are literally screaming at them to pay attention before more serious disease occurs. Yet listening to your body is not just about avoiding future illness. It is about wellness and vitality now and about your being able to have the life you – and your body – will love. I've come to see a person's body intelligence – what we could call your body quotient, or BQ – as a fundamental measure of your health and well-being. Body intelligence is equally important for men, and if you are a male or transgendered person reading this book for yourself or someone you love, welcome! I have many males in my practice, but chose to focus this book on women so that I could speak clearly to women's unique relationships to their bodies. But the principles and practices of being bodywise are just as relevant to males.

As someone who gets migraines, I know the value of pain relief, when we need it, as well as anyone. And yet, patterns of headaches or other kinds of pain can be the body's communication to us about something of value in our lives. After working at a large general practice for 7 years, where I was seeing patients every 15 minutes, I began to consider leaving to open my own holistic practice. Practising medicine with enough time to listen to and honour the hearts of my patients was what I desperately wanted, but I was afraid. I had young children, and I was concerned about the demands of starting a private practice. I had certainly never been trained to run a business, and I was concerned about failing financially and not being able to pay the mortgage or the grocery bills. And, I was also afraid that my more traditional physician colleagues would shun me for practising holistic medicine, which accepts that other healing traditions can have as much efficacy as, and at times more than, Western medicine. There is now a lot of research that demonstrates which complementary treatments work, and which don't, but at the time, this was all very new. So, I delayed leaving. And, as I became increasingly frustrated with my inability to give my patients the kind of care they needed, I began to get neck pain for the first time since my medical internship, and migraine headaches for the first time in my life.

I initially thought that the headaches arose from the neck pain and tried a course of physiotherapy. The therapy helped with the neck pain, but not with the headaches. It took my kind and talented osteopathic colleague – who was treating me for neck pain – to whisper in my ear, 'You know, it's interesting that you only get headaches on your workdays, not when you're home with your kids.' Hmmm. I began to realize that my body was trying to tell me something important. After much reflection and hand-wringing, I came to the difficult conclusion that I needed to leave my job to preserve my own well-being. I had stayed in a work situation that drained me physically and emotionally and was feeling fatigued and depressed. This was my body speaking to me.

Finally, despite my fears, I listened to my body wisdom and resigned from my job. Interestingly, even though my contract required that I continue to work in my position for another 6 months, my migraine headaches completely disappeared. My body wisdom helped me – in fact, forced me! – to transition to the necessary next phase of my healing journey.

Now, as a holistic doctor in private practice, I have never enjoyed being a physician more than I do today. Instead of draining me, my work fulfils, challenges, and inspires me. If I arrive at work in a bad mood, I leave in a good mood, uplifted by my incredible colleagues and the profound healing I get to witness in my patients.

Our symptoms are simply our bodies trying to tell us what they need. We tend to pathologize and medicate the very signals that our bodies send us to direct us toward health. These symptoms are not annoyances that we need to numb or just outright ignore, they are important messages that we can use to seek our own wellness. I help my patients listen to the language of their bodies and, together, we treat the underlying causes of their symptoms, so they can avoid more serious disease and discover real, lasting health.

I live and practise medicine in the US, and particularly, in sunny California. You will notice that some of the terms and references that I use are necessarily based on the US healthcare system, such as it is. But all of the medical information and the bodywise practices are universal, for both women and men, and are as applicable in South Africa as they are in the UK (two of my favourite places). Most of the supplements that I recommend are widely available at your local health shop. And if you can't find them there, take a look online. Just be sure to get them from a reputable supplier (Appendix A is helpful with this!).

The Most Powerful Diagnostic Tool

The most powerful diagnostic tool I have in the treatment room is a woman's own body intelligence. I often say that we will order tests, but that the best test I have is her insight about her own body – what she feels and why, when she is likely to feel that way, what makes her symptoms better or worse. Listening to what she knows about her experience is the key to unlocking the puzzle that causes her pain or suffering. When my patients pay attention to this natural intuition, the results can be quite extraordinary. They were for Sofia. A vivacious, petite woman in her mid-twenties with curly blonde hair, Sofia came into my office carrying her adorable toddler daughter. She laughed easily with her, and their mutual affection was apparent as they played with blocks on the waiting room floor.

Sofia and her husband met and fell in love in their early twenties and were excited about building a home and family. Sofia loved to garden and cook. Creating a healthy home was what truly made her happy. I found myself surprised when I asked her what brought her in and, unexpectedly, she said, 'I'm really afraid that I'm never going to have another child.' At first, I did not understand her fear since, at just 26 years old, there was no reason that she should not be able to have another child. But then she continued, 'I'm having recurrent dreams that a snake is biting me in the head and in the neck, and I'm terrified that something's terribly wrong with me.' I believe in listening very carefully to my patients, and I certainly respect the power of dreams and of the unconscious mind. Yet, to be honest, I did not know what to make of her fear and foreboding.

Sofia was feeling tired to an extent that was unusual even for being the busy mother of a young child. She also was experiencing body aches, so I ordered a number of blood tests. The tests revealed that her thyroid function was low and her blood calcium was high. After further lab tests and brain-imaging studies, we found that Sofia had multiple endocrine neoplasia, which is a syndrome of cancers in many endocrine organs. She had a tumour in her pituitary gland in her brain and another in her parathyroid gland in her neck – just as her dream had foretold. And all of the tumours had made her infertile. We arranged special treatments for her condition and helped her emotionally to deal with this devastating news. The bright spot for Sofia was that because of her body wisdom, she was diagnosed with this condition very early, before any of the cancers could endanger her life. And her father was subsequently diagnosed – and effectively treated – as well.

Although Sofia was unable to have more kids, her body wisdom saved her life and her father's life. She continued to have exquisite intuition about her own body and her own needs throughout the treatment process, helping us as her doctors to help her thrive despite her diagnosis. After her treatment and recovery, Sofia opened a child-care facility in her home and continued to have a fulfilling life, doing what she loved most, which was nurturing and teaching children. She remained healthy and cancer-free, with careful follow-up.

> Becoming bodywise means discovering a new way of being in which you can know what you need, when you need it – and trust yourself to honour those beautiful needs. This is a simple and endlessly adaptable recipe for wellness.

The journey to becoming bodywise is open to all of us, and I want to help you develop the body wisdom you need to thrive. This book is not actually about doing less, because most of my patients don't want to do less. They love their families, and their work, and their lives, and they don't really want to sacrifice any of it. I believe that the answer to good health is not to deny yourself what you love or to try to seek some imaginary life balance. Getting healthy is also not about adding more things to your to-do list. It's not about following a specific diet or exercise programme, because the truth is that every woman's body is unique and needs different things to be healthy.

Rather than some universal prescription for all women, I will offer you the principles and practices that can support you in having the unique and vibrant life that you long for. I am going to teach you how to listen to your body so that you can better understand its messages, when something in your life needs to change. Becoming bodywise means discovering a new way of being in which you can know what you need, when you need it – and trust yourself to honour those beautiful needs. This is a simple and endlessly adaptable recipe for wellness.

As a doctor, a wife, and a mother of three, people ask me all the time, 'How do you do it all and stay healthy?' First, I have to tell you that my health is not perfect. I get sick like everyone else. I have neck pain that flares up when I am stressed or not strengthening or stretching my body enough. I cannot tell you how grateful I am to have an extraordinary chiropractor and acupuncturist in my office. I get migraines with my menstrual cycle. And I have a tendency to have elevated blood sugar, from both hormonal and genetic causes (not to mention the Frosties and Doritos I grew up eating). Sometimes I do too much and compensate by drinking too much really fabulous coffee, which leads to my getting irritable and overtired.

But what brings me back and helps me to heal is being bodywise. My life, like everyone else's, is changing on a daily, weekly, and yearly basis. No static idea of 'balance' has ever worked for me. I am, like all women, constantly trading off time with my beloveds with time to work, exercise, and just to rest and relax. All of us are managing competing needs, our own and others', but being bodywise allows us to navigate our well-being in the changing circumstances of life.

What's Your BQ?

I've long noticed that many of my 40-year-old patients look and feel 60, and that many of my 60-year-old patients look and feel 40. Once I started seeing my patients through the lens of their own body wisdom, it began to make sense. Women who look and feel younger are responsive to the messages they receive from their bodies, which guides their decisions and gives them the kind of ageless beauty that only good health brings. Bodywise women can read their bodies' signals and symptoms and have a felt sense of what they need to be well from year to year, month to month, and even moment to moment. But most important, they honour their knowing with doing. I'll give you one example.

Over the years, I have learned that listening to my body is the fastest way to get the life I want. When I was on call in the emergency room as a medical resident, working 100 hours a week while pregnant with twin girls, there was rarely time to pee or eat – in a system, ironically, that did not honour the health of the very practitioners who were trying to heal people. Not surprisingly, I almost suffered from premature labour and ended up on bed rest for nearly 3 months.

I had taken care of premature babies in the NICU (neonatal intensive care unit) and desperately wanted to do everything I could to protect my daughters' health. My body demanded the rest that I had simply not been giving it. Every week on bed rest, my husband and I celebrated the development that was going on in utero: This week we finally reached nervous-system development. This week we got lung maturity. At the end of my bed rest, I was lucky to have healthy, happy twin girls (6 pounds, 2 ounces, and 6 pounds, 12 ounces!). And all three of us benefited – bed rest probably saved my daughters from being born prematurely. My 4-year-old son also benefited. He loved all of the extra quality time we suddenly got together, being able to cuddle up with me to read a book . . . or a dozen.

We all need to listen to the sometimes-very-clear signals that our bodies are giving us, which we too often ignore.

The Necessity of Becoming BodyWise

I always ask patients to come to their first visit with whatever medications and supplements they are taking so that I can see what is truly worth their time and money and make sure that nothing they are taking is harmful or contraindicated with anything else they are taking. I have patients walk in with literally bags of medicines, vitamins, and herbs. Some people are taking as many as 50 different supplements. And equally worrying, I see people who are taking 25 different prescription drugs. I'm not sure which scares me more. They both can be quite harmful and certainly mask the body's own intelligence. If you're taking a medication or supplement to make you more energetic – how do you know when your body is really tired? And if you are on constant ibuprofen for that neck pain, how would you know whether your poor posture at the computer is hurting you? One of my patients told me that her other doctor gave her Prilosec (Losec) for her reflux and told her that she no longer needed to worry about drinking coffee in the morning and wine before bed, or her exceedingly stressful job that made her feel like she needed to drink both. Something is very wrong with this perspective. Of course, we want to relieve symptoms, but not at the risk of exacerbating the underlying cause.

I am grateful for medicine when it is needed and for supplements that really work, often with fewer side effects than pharmaceuticals, but when you're taking handfuls of pills to feel well, girl, you are really missing something. There is a fundamental problem that is not being addressed, or it wouldn't take so much biochemical experimentation to help you feel better.

Becoming bodywise gives you a basis on which to judge whether a particular vitamin or that antidepressant is really helping you or not. And having a felt sense of which situations or reactions raise or lower your blood pressure gives you better tools to keep your blood pressure in check naturally. I'm in favour of taking medications or supplements that are truly helping or protecting you, but, often, my patients can find healthy ways to reduce their need for chemical help by sensing and taking charge of their bodies' reactions. And lowering your blood pressure by deep breathing or meditation – or even a healthy swearing session inside your closed car – has fewer side effects than any pill.

As I said, I'm not opposed to taking medication when you need it, but my preference is that my patients heal themselves using their body intelligence and their lifestyle choices when possible. That is real, lasting healing and not just symptom relief. It's a healing of the whole body. I have many patients who have dropped their cholesterol levels by as much as 100 points, have reversed diabetes, have ended chronic back pain, and have stopped menopausal hot flushes all by paying attention to their bodies' needs and making lifestyle changes.

No one but you can possibly know what your body needs. Not even your doctor. The practice of medicine is based on research studies that show what makes the average person ill and what therapies can help her or him get better. And 'average' is certainly weighted in the last 50 years toward white male study participants. But even in studies designed for a diverse range of women, 'average' results may or may not apply to you. You are genetically unique, as is your life experience, which we now know dramatically affects the expression of your genes. We no longer live in a time of one-size-fits-all medicine. We sequenced the human genome over a decade ago, and we are now able to measure the incredible diversity of human physiological activity. When one of my patients says, 'I'm sensitive,' I absolutely believe her. Medicines do not affect all people in the same way because our bodies' systems are not all the same.

Don't you know someone who can drink coffee just before bed with no problem? And some of us, like me, cannot drink caffeine after noon without being up until 2:00 a.m.! That is because some of us are fast metabolizers of caffeine, making the effect minimal, and others are genetically slow metabolizers of caffeine, making the caffeine effect longer and more significant. We could do the genetic test that differentiates these two groups of people, but laboratory tests are often unnecessary when juxtaposed with the intuitive awareness of our bodies. Someone who is bodywise is well aware of whether she can happily order a cappuccino at dinner or needs to make it a decaf.

Inside each one of us, right now, is an innate wisdom that can give us specific feedback on how life affects us – from the medicines we take, to the food we eat, to the work we do, to the relationships we have. We need to pay close attention to the clues that our bodies give us to navigate our health and health care.

Even a fantastic clinician – and there are many wonderful doctors and other practitioners – cannot, in 10 minutes, really understand deeply, or help *you* understand deeply, what you need to do in order to be well. He can diagnose common problems like urinary tract infections or sprained ankles, but it's just not enough time to help you make broad changes that will lead to your long-term health and wellness. With doctors ever more pressed for time, it has never been more important for you to be bodywise about what helps you feel well, what makes you feel sick, and what you need to thrive in your life.

I run a clinic where I practise with a naturopath, a chiropractor, an acupuncturist, a psychologist, and other allied professionals. I have deep respect and appreciation for these other healing traditions and how they are able to help patients, often in ways that are complementary to modern medicine. And in many cases, these traditions can help patients where the medical treatments are dangerous or ineffective. And even then, these practitioners cannot know what is happening in your body nearly as well as you can. It is a great blessing to find practitioners you trust, but you never want to hand over the responsibility of your health to another person, no matter how kind or talented she or he is. When any practitioner asks you to take a medication or supplement, listen closely to how your body feels – is this substance improving your health in a way that you can sense or measure? When you allow your intuition to have a voice in decision making, you can avoid taking chemicals, even natural ones, that are not really helping you.

Healing Ourselves, Healing the Earth

We are all born with a deep knowledge of our bodies and their needs. We could not have survived and evolved without it. Before the last century, when we were trying to find food, to survive the elements, and to give birth to and raise children, if we didn't listen to our deep bodily intelligence, we would have died. Yet today, we are living in a world that has never been more removed from our basic physical needs. We can sit at a computer without speaking or moving for an entire day. We rarely grow or gather our own food; with the proliferation of frozen meals and delivery services, we don't even need to cook it. We can take something to help us stay awake all night and take something else to sleep during the day if we want or if our work demands it. Essentially, we can ignore our bodies' needs or signals most of the time and still survive. Eighty per cent of the diseases in developed societies are made far worse, or even caused by our 21st-century lifestyle, including heart disease, high cholesterol, diabetes, and many cancers. Our lack of body wisdom under such conditions is making us sick as a society and as individuals.

I am passionate about helping women to become bodywise because I actually think it is the most powerful and revolutionary way to heal not just ourselves but our society as well. As you will see, when we honour ourselves and our health as women, we end up healing our families, our organizations, and even our relationship to the earth.

When you listen to the voice of your body that's been speaking to you your whole life, and you begin to understand your body's language, you unlock the key to your own happiness and well-being. Decisions that were difficult become simpler. Eating becomes more of a pleasure as you understand what your body really wants. A new level of energy and inspiration is possible when you move, eat, and rest in the way your body needs. You develop a 'second sense' for choosing people who are positive influences, with your body intelligence as your talisman. You are less likely to become ill, as you listen to the early symptoms that your body is communicating to you. And you have the power and potential to heal your own symptoms of chronic body depletion. If you want to have joy and vitality and longevity, begin listening to your natural body wisdom and move from depletion to repletion – to a state of wholeness and full health.

PART ONE

How Do You Become BodyWise?

CHAPTER 1

How Do You Measure and Improve Your BQ?

If you're anything like me, you weren't brought up with the idea that you needed to master and maintain body intelligence, your BQ, along with reading, writing, and arithmetic. You could argue that, in most cultures, mastering the art of *ignoring* your body's needs in the service of 'getting important things done' is part of maturing. And, of course, it is important to be able to delay physical gratification and do little things like provide food and shelter for oneself. But in our societal training, most of us have lost touch with a whole universe of inner knowing that can guide our lives in a healthier direction and create a lot more joy and fun – and who doesn't want that?

Understanding Body Wisdom

Becoming bodywise consists of developing body intelligence at four different levels. I think of this as gathering information about our well-being from the outside-in. First, we gather measurements of our health using data we can collect, often using diagnostic tests or devices to do so. Second, we pay attention to our sensations within our bodies. Third, we track any feelings or emotions that are associated with those sensations. And fourth, we try to discern patterns of experience that help us understand what we sense and feel. Think of the fourth level of discernment as the detective level – combining all of our gathered data, sensations, and emotions and using those clues to lead us to broader insights about our health and well-being.

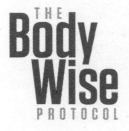

THE Body Wise PROTOCOL

1. **MEASURE:** Gather measured observations of health
2. **SENSE:** Attend to body sensations
3. **FEEL:** Note feelings or intuitions about your body
4. **DISCERN:** Look for patterns of experience that are trying to tell you something, including those influenced by the unconscious mind (dreams, visions, symbols)

Measure

Several years ago, Joe, one of the sweetest, most soft-spoken men I have ever met, walked into my office with a complaint of daily headaches. Unbeknownst to Joe, his blood pressure was 200/120 (normal being 135/85 or less). Joe's headaches were from the pounding blood in his head. And the blood tests we ordered showed that his cholesterol and inflammatory markers were extremely elevated. Joe was a walking time bomb. We got busy on all fronts – stress reduction, exercise, diet changes, and blood pressure medication. Joe is now 20 pounds lighter and an exercise fanatic, with great cholesterol, normal inflammatory markers, and normal blood pressure (on good medication). And, of course, no further headaches. Measuring Joe's health parameters literally saved his life.

In Joe's case, his head could 'sense' his high blood pressure, but, in most cases, we feel nothing when our blood pressure or pulse is high, which is why we need to have it measured occasionally. Paul, on the other hand, came to see me because he *had* measured his blood pressure, and it was high. The mystery was that Paul ate about as healthy a diet as anyone can, was a normal weight, exercised regularly, and had no family history of high blood pressure. Paul did not want to take medication, so we tried supplements, stress reduction, meditation, and more exercise. No luck. We then tried medication. Three different kinds. No luck. His blood pressure was still elevated. Then Paul's wife came into the next visit (I swear this is why married men live longer than single ones) and said, 'You know, honey, I asked you to tell Rachel about your snoring. . . .' Hmmm. Paul was resistant at first to undergoing a medical sleep study – where he would literally sleep in a sleep lab while hooked up to devices to measure oxygen saturation, pulse, and sleep cycles – so we had him use one of the simple devices that tracks sleep cycles at home. The result? He was getting *no* deep sleep. And deep sleep is critical to good health.

A lack of deep sleep can be caused by other issues, but the most common cause is sleep apnoea – literally a stopping of breathing at night. Since not breathing for more than 5 minutes is incompatible with life, the sleeper's body wakes him or her up after a few minutes of apnoea, or no breathing. This cycle continues all night long, with snoring leading to apnoea, and the body awakening the sleeper after a short period of apnoea. This can happen every 6 minutes all night long. The long-term effects of sleep apnoea include daytime sleepiness, less ability to concentrate, depression, and, you guessed it, high blood pressure and significantly increased risk of heart attack.

After his poor sleep results with his home device, Paul was willing to have an official sleep study done, which, in fact, showed severe sleep apnoea. Since then, Paul has been faithfully using his breathing machine (CPAP – continuous positive airway pressure – which keeps those airways open all night) and has normal blood pressure. Not to mention, he is more energetic and happier.

Sometimes a little data collection (blood pressure, sleep-cycle tracking, sleep study) is just what you need to understand what your body is trying to communicate. With just a little help, you can obtain measured observations of your health: blood pressure and pulse, blood oxygen levels, blood sugar, cholesterol levels, weight and body composition, steps taken per day, sleep cycles, and other assessable parameters. Personal health-assessment tools are easily available, such as simply taking your pulse or stepping on the scale to measure your weight or body composition. Using some of the new health-tracking devices, often worn as wristbands or smartwatches, allows us to measure pulse, steps taken per day, exercise duration, or sleep cycles. These devices provide a whole new way to assess our health on an ongoing basis, and even track it online, or compare it with friends'. Medical assessments using blood pressure cuffs, blood and urine laboratory testing, and body composition testing (assessing how much body fat, cellular hydration, and lean tissue you have) are important general measurements of wellness. And even more advanced medical testing is available for assessing cancer risk or cardiovascular risk, for example. It is safe to say that we have never had access to such a wide array of devices and testing to help us understand our health and well-being. We will discuss a number of these devices and give recommendations in Chapter 2. When we combine this factual knowledge with a practised intuition about our well-being, we are much more capable of staying healthy.

Sense

After collecting good data about your wellness from the outside, you need to turn your attention inside your body. The simplest form of your inner knowing is becoming aware of basic body sensations that are signals of your body's well-being: sleepiness, hunger, thirst, muscle fatigue, light-headedness, the need to use the bathroom, pain of various types, sexual desire, and so on. Some of these are easy to interpret: for example, thirst means you need to drink more. Sometimes, it's a bit more complicated. For example, you could feel sleepy because you need more sleep or because your blood sugar is low and you need to eat, or because you are thoroughly bored in your afternoon meeting. When we really start to pay attention to our body signals, we can gain a more nuanced understanding of how our body wants to be cared for.

To some of you, this may sound strange, but not all of us can easily feel our body sensations. It's not that the body isn't 'talking' – but some of us have turned down our brain's receptiveness to body sensation, and simply aren't 'listening.' This is true for the classic stoic person, who is impervious to pain or hunger. We are all stoic from time to time, but for some of us, it becomes a habit – a dangerous one. For example, the women I care for who eat compulsively to satisfy emotional needs (and don't we all from time to time?) can lose their ability to feel the sensation of being full. Without that sensation, overeating becomes the norm, as there is no satiety stop sign to keep us from polishing off that plate of nachos.

When I met Tamar, she was a very successful businesswoman who cried in my office about her inability to control her appetite and her weight. Tamar knew, like we all do, that being overweight was hard on her body, and she was already on the verge of developing diabetes. But she had stressful work and a habit of eating to help her feel calm and safe. Tamar had a history of sexual abuse as a young child and teen. This horrible experience is, unfortunately, not uncommon, with worldwide and US prevalence of sexual abuse ranging from 1 in 4 to 1 in 5 young women under the age of 18.[1] When we are victims of abuse, sexual or otherwise, it is common to psychically 'remove ourselves' – to exit the painful body experience of the abuse by blocking the sensations and absenting our consciousness. Our bodies may be present, but 'we' are not. As a result of this, many women who have experienced trauma develop a habit of being absent from physical sensation, either painful or pleasurable. The numbness to body sensation that started as a defence mechanism can actually endanger the health and enjoyment of the surviving adult. In Tamar's case, she truly could not sense when her stomach was full.

Many of us have periods of our busy lives where we ignore our body's sensations. Certainly I was encouraged in medical school to ignore the need to sleep, eat, pee, or basically do anything other than care for patients or study. I remember a well-known female liver transplant surgeon at my medical school who refused to 'scrub out' of surgery even though her waters broke and she was about to give birth. God bless her, but talk about having to prove yourself and having to ignore your body sensations! Tamar's healing involved learning to 're-inhabit' her body and to identify and sense what was going on inside her – along with feeling the emotions that those sensations evoked. I referred Tamar to a trained trauma therapist to assist her in this process and to create a safe place where Tamar could heal, and learn to feel again. The therapist led Tamar in exercises where she reclaimed her own physical body and boundaries, and by focusing her attention inside her body, she began to sense her body sensations again. Peter Levine, PhD, is a psychologist and author who founded a school of trauma therapy, Sensory Awareness, that focuses on helping people restore their perception of the many sensations of the body. If you have had any kind of trauma, his books and the therapists trained in his methods are a valuable resource (see Appendix B).

Tamar was ultimately able to experience the sensations of her stomach being full. The impact was huge. Tamar gradually lost more than 50 pounds over 2 years, reversed her pre-diabetes, and felt so much better in her body. And for the first time in her life, she was able to really experience not only the pleasure of eating, but sexual pleasure as well. She felt like a new, and whole, woman.

Feel

In this step, we can begin to turn our attention even deeper inward and note the emotions that arise in association with our body's sensations. A few years ago, I had a discussion with one of my healthy patients in her mid-forties about whether or not to get a mammogram. The recommendation at the time was to do mammography screenings every 2 years between age 40 and 50 (currently, they are not necessarily recommended *at all* between age 40 and 50). She'd had a mammogram the year before, so I let her know that she didn't have to have one again this year, but that it was her decision. She said that she felt an intense pull in her gut as we discussed it, and, when she really felt into it, the sensation in her gut was fear. She didn't know why, but she felt compelled to get another mammogram, so I agreed and referred her. With that mammogram, she was diagnosed with the earliest possible grade of breast cancer, and she was able to be cancer-free with a lumpectomy. Her 'gut feeling' literally saved her life.

Our 'feeling intelligence' can save our lives. It helps us pick wonderful partners or spouses. It guides us to say what a potential client needs to hear to clinch the deal, or intuits when our children are truly ill as opposed to wanting to skip their oral history presentations. Our feeling brain is the staunch ally of our well-being, if we can 'feel' it and act upon what we're told.

In my office, there are multiple courses of action that may work for each patient, and I try to draw out of my patients which course *they* think will be most successful for them. They, therefore, get to take ownership of their own health care, and, because they *intuit* that this is the right course for them, it is much more likely to be successful. Keep in mind that the placebo effect – really our bodies' ability to heal themselves – is 30 per cent, and even as high as 40 per cent, with any treatment.[2] I want to engage my patients' inner healing abilities, so I need their 'gut feelings' to lead us in our treatments.

Our thinking and feeling abilities are present throughout our entire bodies. We have extensive plexuses of neurons around our hearts and around our intestines that moderate and guide our emotional responses. This emotional body intelligence is reflected in expressions like our 'heart's desire' and our 'gut feelings.' In fact, HeartMath Institute in Boulder Creek, California, has demonstrated that our 'heart thinking' and intuition precede our 'in the skull' thinking and intuition in much of our predictive decision-making.[3]

These nerve plexuses around the gut and heart are part of our sympathetic and parasympathetic nervous system and therefore directly linked up with our fight-or-flight stress response. This ability to 'feel' what we are thinking is fundamental to our survival skills. A woman walking down a dark street at night is hyperaware of her surroundings (the sense level of body intelligence) and is also paying attention to the feelings of her heart and her gut intuition (related to a feeling in her belly or a squeezing of her chest that she associates with fear). In only a few seconds, she puts together all of these body signals into a pattern she knows means danger (discernment) that instructs her to cross the street or hail a taxi, rather than continue on her way. These emotional 'hunches' are what kept us safe in the jungles and still keep us safe in the 'jungles' of our current lives.

As an example of how you might access your body-feeling intelligence, I want to teach you an exercise that I first learned from Julie Schwartz Gottman, PhD, a brilliant psychologist and bodywise woman in her own right. The intention is to use your body as your divination tool to understand what you intuitively know – on the inside.

Luckily for us, we can actually use our bodies as tuning forks for truth – our unique tool to understand our bodies' intelligence. When one strikes a tuning fork of a particular musical note, and then brings it near a tuning fork of the same note, the second tuning fork begins to vibrate and 'sing' – even though it hasn't been struck. It recognizes and senses the vibration of the other tuning fork. This exercise helps your body recognize and sing the musical note of 'yes' for an idea or concept that you feel alignment with – and to produce a discordant note when you do not feel in alignment.

Exercise 1: Tuning In to Your 'Yes' and 'No'

1. Sit comfortably and take three deep breaths to relax and be present in your body. If you would like, close your eyes.

2. Imagine an untruth, for example, 'I hate kittens' or 'I hate roses.' Repeat this statement over and over again to yourself. As in the 'Quality of Sensation' exercise on page 32, observe the sensations in as much detail as you can. You may feel tightness in your chest, heaviness on your shoulders, a knot in the pit of your stomach, shaking in your hands, coldness in your feet, or a lack of any sensation. Observe the sensations in as much detail as you can. Note the type of sensation (pressure, stabbing, aching) and its size, density, temperature, or colour. What you feel in your body is the 'No' of your body intelligence. It's the sensation of your body reacting to and rejecting this untruth.

3. Then reverse what you've just said to yourself, repeating the true statement to yourself next, like 'I love roses' or 'I adore kittens.' Then, see how your body responds. What does your body feel when you've now spoken your own truth? You might feel warmth and opening in your chest or a tingling in your belly, arms, or legs, or a smile or softness around your eyes. Note the type of sensation (tingling, airy, expansive) and its size, density, temperature, or colour. This difference in internal body sensation is your gauge of truth, your body's way of telling you what is true for you and what is not. What you feel in your body is the 'Yes' of your body intelligence. It's the sensation of your body fully opening to that possibility.

4. Now, take three more deep breaths and then open your eyes.

For this exercise, find a comfortable place to sit that is free from distractions. If you have trouble feeling your body sensations, do not worry! We will be learning how to do that, in detail, in Chapter 2. You can listen to a recording of this exercise at doctorrachel.com.

This exercise can help you sense your body's own version of 'yes' and 'no' in any situation. With practice, you can learn to interpret your body's language – the meaning of each of those sensations in the current moment – in order to make decisions for your benefit.

Discern

When I realized that I only had migraines on my workdays (I worked part-time) and not on the other days of the week, it became clear (with a little help from my osteopath) that this pattern of migraines was my body telling me that my job was literally 'a headache.' And when I listened to my body intelligence and quit my job, my headaches disappeared. I am frequently searching for these patterns of body wisdom in the stories of my patients in order to help them navigate their wellness. I have had at least six patients in my practice who complained of various kinds of gynaecological issues – pain with sex, chronic pelvic pain, recurrent bladder infections – and experienced spontaneous healing of their issues when they left the dysfunctional relationship they were in.

Scientific studies are increasingly demonstrating how much the unconscious brain directs our lives. The 'unconscious' is like the enormous iceberg that is under the water, showing only the tip of itself to conscious awareness. This means that the huge majority of sensory information that we are exposed to – from both inside and outside the body – is processed by the unconscious mind. This is how seemingly magical experiences – like my patient Sofia (see page xiv) who dreamed of her cancer before it was diagnosed – occur. The unconscious mind – active in the background all along – brings something to consciousness in a dream or vision that informs you of what is happening in your body and in your life. It is possible to use the unconscious mind for your benefit by becoming aware of patterns of experience that may be trying to tell you something.

One of the ways that the unconscious helps us is by linking current experiences to memorable experiences from our past. For example, in the section above, when we discussed the woman walking down a dark street at night, you can bet your life that if she had been mugged or assaulted in a similar situation in the past, her warning signs (heart rate, blood pressure, chest or belly sensations) would be activating off the charts, as opposed to giving her subtle suggestions. Our unconscious is trying to protect us from danger, and figuring out *why* we feel the way we feel is an important part of discernment. For example, my mother bakes the most outrageously delicious cinnamon sticky buns you have ever had in your life. They generally arrived in my childhood home, hot out of the oven and steaming with their doughy, caramel nuttiness, at Christmas (presents!) or when the family were all at home cosily celebrating Thanksgiving (warmth, comfort, love, safety).

Through my powers of discernment, I am able to understand why I have a hard time walking past a cinnamon bun bakery without actively salivating on the floor. All of those sweet emotional experiences associated with cinnamon and caramel baked goods make it very tempting for me to stop in for a snack whenever I smell them. But what I really want when I get a craving for cinnamon buns has a lot more to do with my memories than my hunger, and being able to discern the difference between those two longings is a key to becoming bodywise.

Measuring Your BQ

Now that you understand the four levels of body wisdom, just how bodywise are you? I have developed a quiz to test your BQ, your body intelligence quotient, so that you have an idea of where you're starting on the road to becoming bodywise. I want to give you a place to start in your quest, so that you know where you need to focus your attention to improve your BQ. And by improving your BQ, you can dramatically improve your overall well-being. Take this brief quiz now, and be honest. You don't need to share it with anyone else unless you want to. I'm going to have you repeat it again at the end of the book, to see if you've been able to raise your BQ. And if you do well on this test, wonderful! You can use your bodywise talent to understand and implement all of the ideas to improve your health and your symptoms throughout the course of this book.

BQ Quiz
Measure

1. Do you know your average blood pressure over the past 2 years?

1	2	3	4	5
(I can't ever remember taking it!)		(I'm pretty sure it's okay)	(I know the range within 10 points)	

2. Do you know your weight within 5 pounds? (If you avoid checking your weight because checking it has a negative impact on you, but stay in a stable range, give yourself a 4 or 5.)

1	2	3	4	5
(I don't know it within 15 pounds)		(I know it within 10 pounds)	(I am aware of typical weekly or monthly fluctuations in my weight)	

3. If you are older than 45, do you know if your cholesterol is excellent, average, or too high? (If you are younger than 45, give yourself a 5 – unless you *know* that your family has a history of high cholesterol and haven't measured it.)

1	2	3	4	5
(I've never measured it)		(I've measured it, but I am not sure if it's normal)	(I know the general number and whether it's normal)	

(continued)

BQ Quiz *(cont.)*

4. If you are older than 45, do you know what your fasting blood sugar is? (If you are younger than 45, give yourself a 5 – unless you *know* that your family has a history of diabetes and haven't measured it.)

1	2	3	4	5
(I've never measured it)		(I've measured it, but I am not sure if it's normal)		(I know the general number and whether it's normal)

5. Are you aware of the number of hours of sleep that you get and the quality of your sleep?

1	2	3	4	5
(I have no clue)		(If you give me a few hours, I could figure it out)		(I know how much sleep I get and how much I need)

6. What is or was your average menstrual cycle length (the time from one period to the next)? (If you have never had a menstrual cycle, give yourself a 5.)

1	2	3	4	5
(What is a menstrual cycle?)		(I have a vague sense of when I might bleed)		(I've always known the length of my regular or irregular cycle)

7. Are you aware of when you ovulate? (Or if you don't ovulate, did you used to know when you ovulated?) If you know you've never ovulated, give yourself a 4 or 5.

1	2	3	4	5
(What is ovulation?)		(I have a vague sense of when I might ovulate)		(I always know the day that I ovulate)

Subtotal for Measure: _____
(Add each of your 7 scores together.)

Sense

1. When eating a meal, are you aware of when you are full prior to becoming 'stuffed'?

1	2	3	4	5
(Never)	(Rarely)	(Sometimes)	(Usually)	(Almost always)

2. Do you stop eating before becoming 'stuffed'?

1	2	3	4	5
(Never)	(Rarely)	(Sometimes)	(Usually)	(Almost always)

3. Do you have a snack or meal within 30 minutes of feeling hunger pangs?

1	2	3	4	5
(Never)	(Rarely)	(Sometimes)	(Usually)	(Almost always)

4. Do you typically go to the bathroom within 15 minutes of feeling the need to do so?

1	2	3	4	5
(Never)	(Rarely)	(Sometimes)	(Usually)	(Almost always)

5. When you feel pain in your muscles or joints, do you stop activities that exacerbate your pain?

1	2	3	4	5
(Never)	(Rarely)	(Sometimes)	(Usually)	(Almost always)

6. Are you aware when your neck, back, wrists, hands, or legs are tired from repetitive work activities (such as typing, writing, computer work, phone use, or driving)? Alternatively, if you do work that is mostly physical, are you aware when your body needs a break from the physical work in order to avoid pain or injury?

1	2	3	4	5
(Never)	(Rarely)	(Sometimes)	(Usually)	(Almost always)

7. If your work situation allows it, do you take a break from repetitive work to stand, stretch, walk, rest, or otherwise care for your body at least every 90 minutes? (If your work prevents you from doing this, even if you want to, give yourself a 5 – and let's see if we can find you another job.)

1	2	3	4	5
(Never)	(Rarely)	(Sometimes)	(Usually)	(Almost always)

8. In the last year, how often have you experienced the feeling of sexual desire in your body?

1	2	3	4	5
(Never)	(Once a month to once a year)	(Once a week to once a month)	(1–3 times a week)	(More than 3 times a week)

9. Do you find a healthy way to meet your sexual needs (alone or with a partner)?

1	2	3	4	5
(Never)	(Rarely)	(Sometimes)	(Usually)	(Almost always)

Subtotal for Sense: _____
(Add each of your 9 scores together.)

(continued)

BQ Quiz *(cont.)*

Feel

1. In the last 6 months, how often have you had a 'gut feeling' about a decision or a person that turned out to be true?

1	2	3	4	5
(Never)	(2–3 times a year)	(At least once a month)	(Weekly or more)	(Daily)

2. How often do you listen to and follow your 'gut feelings' about a decision or a person?

1	2	3	4	5
(Never)	(Rarely)	(Sometimes)	(Usually)	(Almost always)

3. Close your eyes and take a moment to imagine the future loss of a pet or someone that you love. Can you feel where and how that sensation of loss lives in your body?

1	2	3	4	5
(I can't feel anything)	(Can feel it, but can't describe it)	(Can feel where it is only)	(Can feel the location and intensity)	(Can describe location, quality, intensity, even colour or form of the sensation)

4. Imagine that you have just been told that you are going to receive a large sum of money for something that you have created to share with the world. Can you feel where and how the sensation of excitement or surprise or relief lives in your body?

1	2	3	4	5
(I can't feel anything)	(Can feel it, but can't describe it)	(Can feel where it is only)	(Can feel the location and intensity)	(Can describe location, quality, intensity, even colour or form of the sensation)

Subtotal for Feel: _____
(Add each of your 4 scores together.)

Discern

1. Consider an area of your body that is or has been in pain. Can you identify behaviours (activities, consumption of certain foods, supplements or medications, massage, or acupuncture) that relieve the pain?

1	2	3	4	5
(I can't identify any)		(I can identify at least one behaviour that relieves my pain)		(I can easily identify multiple behaviours that relieve my pain)

2. Can you identify behaviours (activities, consumption of certain foods, or lack of sleep) that worsen your pain?

1	2	3	4	5
(I can't identify any)		(I can identify at least one behaviour that worsens my pain)		(I can easily identify multiple behaviours that worsen my pain)

3. How easy is it to identify an emotional experience that can cause or exacerbate pain in your body (i.e., headache, menstrual pain, neck or back pain, injury)? For example, 'I notice that when I'm under a lot of stress, my period is much more painful.'

1	2	3	4	5
(Impossible)		(I can identify 1–2 emotional experiences that affect my pain)		(I can easily identify multiple emotional experiences that influence my pain)

4. Can you identify emotional experiences (stress relief during holidays, being with someone you love, being cared for) that decrease your experience of pain?

1	2	3	4	5
(I can't identify any)		(I can identify 1–2 emotional experiences that decrease my pain)		(I can easily identify multiple emotional experiences that decrease my pain)

5. Take a moment to remember the last time that you were ill. How easy is it to discern the patterns of behaviour or exposure that contributed to your being ill?

1	2	3	4	5
(I can't identify any)		(I can think of 1–2 behaviours that may have contributed)		(I can easily think of patterns of behaviour that made me vulnerable to becoming ill)

Subtotal for Discern: _____
(Add each of your 5 scores together.)

	EXCELLENT	GOOD	NEED IMPROVEMENT
Subtotal for Measure (range is 7–35): _____	31–35	24–30	<24
Subtotal for Sense (range is 9–45): _____	40–45	32–39	<32
Subtotal for Feel (range is 4–20): _____	18–20	14–17	<14
Subtotal for Discern (range is 5–25): _____	23–25	18–22	<18
TOTAL (range is 25–125): _____	112–125	88–108	<88

> Once you begin to learn your body's language, you will find that she is a clear and effective communicator and 100 per cent on the side of your having the life you really want and deserve. After all, your body *is* you. And when your mind, heart, and body are aligned, it's amazing what miracles can happen in your life.

If you are 'excellent' in all areas, congratulations! This book will help you become fluent in your body language and capable of preventing problems before they arise. You can use your body intelligence to utilize all of the resources and information in this book to create a joyful bodywise life. If you are 'good,' reading the next chapter, in detail, and doing the exercises will help you build the foundation of your body wisdom. If you 'need improvement' in your ability to listen to the language of your body and to care for yourself, this book is the perfect journey to support you on that quest. Even small improvements in your ability to understand what your body is telling you can make a *big* difference in your health and happiness.

I have found, in my own journey of learning the language of my body, that my body is both resilient and forgiving. If I make even small efforts to care for myself (taking a small break from writing this book to stretch my neck and shoulders), my body feels dramatically better (no pain!). And, if I perpetually refuse to listen to my body, my body turns up the volume – like yesterday, when I *didn't* take a break from writing to stretch and then had severe neck pain all evening. Once you begin to learn your body's language, you will find that she is a clear and effective communicator and 100 per cent on the side of your having the life you really want and deserve. After all, your body *is* you. And when your mind, heart, and body are aligned, it's amazing what miracles can happen in your life.

CHAPTER 2

How Do You Build Your Body Intelligence?

mproving your body intelligence quotient, or BQ, is easier than you might think. It all starts with learning the BodyWise Protocol: how to measure, sense, feel, and discern the language of your body. And although your body's language is absolutely unique to you, the basic principles of how to learn and listen to your body are the same for everyone. Here are some suggestions and exercises to help you with each of the four levels. You may want to pay particular attention to the aspects of the BodyWise Protocol that you did *not* score well on in the BQ Quiz on page 11.

Improving Your Ability to Measure

Learning how to collect information about the healthy functioning of your body is perhaps the simplest level of the BodyWise Protocol. This part of body language we understand because it is translated into words and numbers – a human language that we are used to. We'll discuss both simple and high-tech methods by which to measure your body's health on a moment-to-moment basis.

Pulse and Blood Pressure

Let's begin with the basics: measuring your pulse and blood pressure. Measuring your pulse and blood pressure is probably the quickest way to assess your physiology and stress state. And a bodywise woman can *feel* when her pulse is elevated or *hear* when her heart accelerates with excitement or fear.

Your pulse is the regular 'beat' of pressure in your blood vessels that comes from your heart contracting and pushing the blood through your arteries. Your blood pressure is literally the pressure at which your blood is hurtling through your arteries and is measured with two numbers, for example, 130/75. The number on top (systolic blood pressure) is a measure of the highest point of pressure in your arteries. The number on the bottom (diastolic blood pressure) is a measure of the lowest point of pressure in your arteries.

So why is this important? Your heartbeat (or pulse) reflects your body's ability to get blood filled with oxygen and nutrients to the tissues of your body. Both your pulse and blood pressure elevate when the demand for oxygen increases, for example, during exercise. The more physically fit you are, the more efficient your heart muscle and blood vessels are, meaning it takes less pressure to move your blood around. For example, an average 40-year-old woman may have a pulse of 70 beats per minute (bpm), while a 40-year-old female marathon runner can have a normal pulse of 45 bpm.

A relaxed, fit person will generally have a lower pulse and blood pressure. A stressed out, less physically fit person will generally have a higher pulse and blood pressure. Blood pressure can also be impacted by your age, genetics, and medications that you take. That's why it's so important to keep track of your blood pressure regularly: It can alert you to changes that are happening naturally or unnaturally in your body and allow you to take action sooner.

Your blood pressure, especially the top number, or systolic, blood pressure, rises with any real or perceived stress. The body doesn't differentiate between *real* stress (I'm about to be hit by a car) and *perceived* stress (I'm about to purchase my first car). When you are stressed, your body responds as if you are in danger of dying from physical causes – for example, being attacked by a sabre-toothed tiger. It is preparing you to *fight* (stand your ground and take on that tiger) or *flee* (get the hell out of there before you're the tiger's dinner). Your blood vessels dilate in the big muscles of the arms and legs so that you can run for your life and constrict in all nonessential organs (your digestive system or your genitals). This fight-or-flight reaction works beautifully to save you when you are about to get hit by a car – increasing your reaction time and strength. It does not work so well when you are trying to be cool and savvy when *purchasing* your first car.

Measuring your pulse is easy once you get the hang of it. Try putting two fingers on the inside of your wrist below your thumb, and see if you can feel your pulse. Move your fingers around on your wrist until you find the best spot. Try both the right and the left wrists, as it might be easier to feel it on one side than the other. If this is difficult, try feeling for your pulse at your carotid artery (a bigger artery) by lightly pressing two fingers on your neck, below the angle of your jaw. Do not press hard on the carotid artery in the neck as the brain doesn't like it when you cut off its blood supply!

The easiest way to measure your pulse is to count the number of beats for 6 seconds and add a zero to the result. If you want a more accurate assessment of your pulse, count for 30 seconds and multiply by 2. For example, 36 beats in 30 seconds calculates to 72 bpm. The range of a normal pulse in an adult is from 60 to 100 bpm. However, if your pulse is between 45 and 60, you are physically fit, and you do not have issues with lightheadedness, you are probably just fine. Elite-level athletes routinely have a resting pulse between 45 and 55.

> When we breathe deeply, we activate the opposite reactions of the sympathetic nervous system. We slow our pulses, lower our blood pressures, relax our muscles, and send more blood to our digestive systems and genitals.

Counting your pulse is easy if your pulse is regular, meaning that the beats occur approximately the same length of time apart from each other, like a musical drumbeat. Most of us have a regular pulse. It is normal for the pulse to speed up a bit if you are anxious or to slow down if you relax with a few deep breaths. When we breathe deeply, we activate the opposite reactions of the sympathetic nervous system. We slow our pulses, lower our blood pressures, relax our muscles, and send more blood to our digestive systems and genitals.

Some of us have an irregular pulse, meaning that the length of time between beats is not regular. It can feel like we have 'skipped' a beat or multiple beats. The great majority of the time, these irregularities are benign, meaning not dangerous. Some of us can sense them as a 'flutter' or 'flip-flop' in the chest. Almost all of these premature beats are increased in quantity by stress and stimulants. It does happen, however, that sometimes heartbeat irregularities can be dangerous. If your pulse feels irregular to you, it is always best to have it evaluated by your doctor.

Try feeling your pulse while imagining a stressful situation. Does it increase? Now take three long, deep breaths into your belly. Does your pulse slow down? Our pulse rate can measure the basic stress setpoint of our bodies. It is a direct reminder of our ongoing stress levels and our need to slow down and take a few breaths. If you happen to have an electronic activity tracker (such as a chest band heart rate monitor or a wristband that specifically measures heart rate), you can use it to measure your heart rate and its changes.

Measuring blood pressure can involve a little more equipment, but it is still a very easy thing to do. You can purchase an automatic arm blood pressure cuff (the wrist ones don't work as well) and take your own blood pressure at home. There are manual blood pressure cuffs that are very accurate, but require the use of a cuff, a stethoscope, and generally another person in order to listen and observe the pressure readings. There are also a variety of health apps that will help you track your blood pressure, pulse, weight, activity, and other health parameters. Many of them can link directly with your blood pressure cuff. If you're tech savvy, you may want to consider purchasing a blood pressure cuff that can synchronize with an online app and your other electronic activity trackers, if you have them. If you're curious about your blood pressure but don't want to purchase a blood pressure cuff, it is fine to try the blood pressure machines at your local pharmacy. Most of them are fairly accurate.

The reason it can be valuable for you to measure your blood pressure in a relaxed environment is because blood pressure is notoriously elevated at the doctor's office. I don't wear a white coat, but I can tell you that many of my patients, even those that feel very comfortable with me, have dramatically elevated blood pressures in my office and very normal blood pressures at home. They may not *think* that they are stressed when they see me, but their bodies say otherwise! No one wants to be started on blood pressure medication unnecessarily, so if you have had elevated pressures at the doctor's office, I strongly recommend doing some home testing first to get a full picture throughout the day.

Blood pressure, like pulse, varies greatly throughout the day depending on your activity and stress levels. I think it's more useful to think of blood pressure not as a number, but as a range of numbers. At rest, it is ideal to have the top number (systolic blood pressure) lower than 135 and the bottom number (diastolic blood pressure) lower than 85. We define high blood pressure as 140/90 and above. But your cardiac and stroke risk begins to increase for every increment over 115/75 as illustrated in the graph (opposite).

Normal blood pressure can be as low as 85/55, but if you are this low or lower and having symptoms – lightheadedness, nausea, fatigue, blurred vision – please see your doctor! There may be treatment available to help stabilize your blood pressure.

As you get comfortable measuring your own blood pressure, take note of when it is relatively high. This is a good indicator of your body's stress response. How is it at work? After being in rush-hour traffic? After a fight with your loved one? And how effectively can you lower your blood pressure? I mentioned that many of my patients have relatively higher blood pressure when they're in my office. It is also true that most of my patients

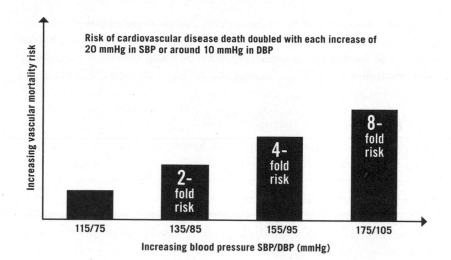

Risk of cardiovascular disease death doubled with each increase of 20 mmHg in SBP or around 10 mmHg in DBP

Increasing vascular mortality risk

2-fold risk

4-fold risk

8-fold risk

115/75   135/85   155/95   175/105

Increasing blood pressure SBP/DBP (mmHg)

can, with three simple, deep breaths, lower their blood pressure levels by as many as 20 points. We have such intimate control over the stress response of our bodies! If you know that your blood pressure rises after stressful work situations, you can protect your heart and brain by taking action to lower it, naturally. Take your pulse (and your blood pressure, if you can) right now. Then try the simple, but surprisingly effective, stress-lowering exercise below. This 5-2-7 breath is an ancient practice that has also been endorsed more recently by Andrew Weil, MD.

Now, measure your pulse (and blood pressure, if you can) again. Did it change? When you become adept at using your breath to relax, you can diffuse tension in even the most trying of circumstances. I have used simple belly breathing to help patients diffuse everything from severe panic attacks in my office to marital conflict. It can literally take the 'fight' out of your

Exercise 2: Belly Breathing

1. Inhale through your nose and exhale through your mouth.
2. Put your hand on your belly and breathe deeply into your abdomen, feeling it push out your hand. This is simple belly breathing.
3. If you want a deeper practice, inhale through your nose to a count of 5, and then pause for a count of 2, feeling the stillness between breaths.
4. Exhale slowly through your mouth to a count of 7, allowing tension to release.
5. Repeat at least five times, or until you feel relaxed.

aggressive fight-or-flight reaction and restore your equanimity, so that you can think clearly and resolve your conflicts, without verbal or physical violence. And being more relaxed and patient can help with your relationships at home and at work.

Weight and Body Composition

It's hard to find a more controversial or hated 'measurement' of a woman's body than weight. Recently, one of my friends and colleagues – a very smart and capable woman – said to me after taking the BQ Quiz: 'Of course, I know my weight. I measure it every morning, and it determines whether I have a good day or a bad day.' This from a beautiful, healthy woman. It is challenging to say anything impactful about women and weight and expect to be heard among the cacophony of negative societal messages. I feel it is my responsibility to guard the mental as well as the physical health of my patients. Which is why I never insist on checking the weights of my patients, if they don't want to be checked. The truth is that I like to know a patient's weight, if it doesn't send her into an emotionally dark place to check it. It is primarily helpful in that, when I see her in another 3 months and she is upset about gaining 10 pounds, I can assure her that, actually, she hasn't.

We women are brutal to ourselves about our weight. And what is weight, anyway? A measure of your gravitational pull. Nothing more, nothing less. There is a decent amount of research showing that a woman who exercises, eats well, and has love in her life is healthy regardless of her weight. I won't say that it's good to be obese or overweight – it is hard on the joints and can increase the risk of diabetes. But I will say that I have *many* women in my practice in the overweight or obese category who have perfect health parameters – blood pressure, cholesterol, blood sugar, in-depth nutritional measurement, strength, and flexibility – who I do not think are at risk in terms of their health. A very thin woman with poor health habits has more health risks than an overweight woman with good health habits. I also have a number of women in my practice who struggle to keep weight on – who are naturally slim, but become dangerously thin when under stress or in challenging circumstances. This is also not easy. And there is very little sympathy for how hard it is on them.

Many health practitioners have abandoned the use of weight alone and now use the BMI (body mass index) to follow their patients. The BMI takes height into account and gives a common scale that is supposed to work for everyone. It doesn't work for extremely muscular people, who may weigh more than is recommended for their height because of their high muscle mass. Having a lot of muscle, of course, can be a very healthy thing, so even the BMI is relative. BMI is a ratio of height divided by weight that is simple in the metric system and a little more complicated in the English system.

BMI = Weight (Kilograms)/Height (Meters)^2

BMI = Weight (Pounds)/Height (Inches)^2 x 703

You can find an explanation for BMI and a BMI calculator at www. nhs.uk/tools/pages/healthyweightcalculator.aspx.

Neither weight nor BMI tells us anything about our body composition – how much water weight, muscle and organ weight, and fat weight we have. For example, I sometimes run group fitness and cleansing programmes in my office. During the last one, after 3 months of *very* good behaviour, I had gained 3 pounds. Which would have been frustrating if I hadn't been measuring my body composition. I had actually lost 7 pounds of fat and a pound of extracellular fluid (the kind you don't want too much of). I gained 9 pounds of muscle and 2 pounds of intracellular fluid (the kind that makes your cells plump and happy). My weight had increased, but so did my health. Less fat, better hydration, more muscle. All good! If measuring your weight puts you in a dark place emotionally, it may not be worth measuring it regularly. I don't necessarily think that all of us benefit from having scales in our bathrooms. However, the average female in the United States gains 5 pounds after the autumn and winter holidays every year. And that's not a genetic thing. That's a cakes, sweets, turkey, and stuffing thing. It's easy to be unconscious about eating if you're not monitoring the impact on your weight or your waistline. It's important to stay accountable to yourself in some way so that you can avoid putting on those pounds. Because taking them off is *so* much more difficult than putting them on. And putting them on year after year is how 35 per cent of the US – and the UK – adult population became obese. We want to be bodywise and learn how to stop the weight-gain march. Part of the key is to be accountable to your body.

Allegra is one of the healthiest patients in my practice. She can inspire you with her intricate knowledge of the strength and flexibility of your body and make you wet your pants laughing at the crazy stories she tells. She, like many of us, had issues with eating and body image as a young woman. Allegra had gained about 20 pounds that she was unhappy about, despite eating pretty well and exercising vigorously. We devised a weight-loss plan for her that worked to shed about 15 of those pounds – all of which were fat by body composition measurement. Recently, she confided in me that she had stopped weighing herself for a few months and gained 6 pounds, eating what anyone would call a healthy diet. Just a little too much of it. She restarted her daily measurements for a week, and just that reminder helped her take off 2 pounds in 4 days. Like many of us, Allegra has a love-hate relationship with the scale. She needs it as a measurement that contributes to her body wisdom and is working hard to see it just as that and not a judgement of her worth.

There are many ways to measure and have body accountability. If you feel good about weighing yourself at home, be sure you have an accurate scale. You can also look for a scale that measures body composition, keeping in mind that these are not perfectly accurate. If you want a more accurate measure of body composition, you'll have to consult a trainer, nutritionist, physiotherapist, or doctor who can perform this for you. Some practitioners still use skin calipers to estimate total body fat by 'pinching' the skin in various locations in your body. More accurate than body composition measured on a scale or with calipers is a bioimpedance analysis (BIA), which can be measured in a practitioner's office in a matter of minutes. It sends an electric current through your body and measures resistance, from which it analyses the amount of fat, lean tissue, and fluid that your body contains. The most accurate measure of body composition is done by personal trainers and doctors using water displacement or air displacement techniques, though these are expensive and take more time.

If you would prefer to never set foot on a scale for the rest of your life, but would like some kind of measure of body fat to remain accountable, another option is to measure the circumference of your waist. If you lose body fat, it is very likely that you will lose some of it around your waist, and you can measure that with a tape measure.

You'll be interested to know that from a health standpoint – risk of heart attack, stroke, and diabetes – fat stored in the thighs and buttock area is not nearly as risky as fat stored in the belly. Belly fat is inflammatory and linked to heart disease, whereas that fine, large butt and thighs of yours do not increase your risk at all. If you would like specific directions on how to measure your waist and hip circumference, these can be found in Appendix A.

Tracking Your Menstrual Cycle

Our menstrual cycles depend on hormones from our pituitary glands (luteinizing hormone, LH, and follicle-stimulating hormone, FSH) 'talking' to our ovaries. Under that hormonal influence, the ovaries then produce an egg, which, if unfertilized by a sperm, sheds along with the uterine lining approximately 2 weeks later, creating menstrual bleeding. This sequence of events is the female menstrual cycle, with fluctuating hormones (oestrogen, progesterone, and testosterone) shifting throughout and keeping the rhythm of the cycle itself. There are a number of women who are not under the influence of these hormonal fluctuations.

- Women on the birth control pill, patch, ring, implant, or injection who have suppressed ovulation (the release of an egg) and therefore only bleed after withdrawal of the hormones
- Women who have gone through menopause and no longer menstruate
- Women who are pregnant
- Women who don't menstruate for medical reasons (i.e., polycystic ovarian syndrome, low or high thyroid function, extremely low weight or body fat, or others)
- Women who have had their ovaries removed or have had chemotherapy or radiation that has stopped ovarian function
- Young women who haven't gone through menarche yet (haven't had their first period)

For those of you who are still menstruating, even if your cycle is irregular, you are influenced by the hormonal milieu of the part of the cycle that you are in – perhaps more than you realize. Your mood, hunger, emotional stability, sexual drive, tendency to headache, and breast size and tenderness are just a few of the experiences that fluctuate with your cycle. If you have never tracked your cycle, I would strongly encourage you to do so. Not only can you avoid pregnancy more effectively (if you need to) and get pregnant more easily (if you want to) but you can also anticipate and understand your own physical and emotional fluctuations in a whole new way. Some of the physical changes that track with your cycle include:

- Basal body temperature: Your basal temperature peaks at ovulation and stays high for the last half of the cycle. To measure it, use a very sensitive thermometer when you wake in the morning.
- Breast tenderness: This can start at ovulation, but breasts definitely tend to swell in the week or two before your period.
- Cervical mucus: I know . . . *what*??? Literally, cervical mucus is the liquid that comes out of your cervix. Your cervix is the bottom of your uterus (where a baby could grow and where your menstrual blood comes from) and can be felt deep in the vagina (it feels firm, but flexible, like the end of your nose). You can check cervical fluid by just looking in your underwear, as it flows out of your vagina, or you can insert a finger into your vagina and draw out the fluid and check it out. At ovulation, the fluid is clear and viscous, like egg white, allowing the sperm to swim to their target. During the rest of your cycle, the cervical mucus is white and thin.

Probably the easiest way to track your symptoms these days is with a smartphone or computer app designed for that purpose. There are many. Or, you can do it the old-school way on a chart made for that purpose. You can find a chart for that purpose at doctorrachel.com under the BodyWise tab. If you are looking for guidance and more detail on how to understand your cycle, the book *Taking Charge of Your Fertility* is a wonderful guide.[1]

Tracking your cycle and understanding its influence on your life is a fundamental advantage of being a bodywise woman. It allows you to avoid scheduling that ultra-important event in the grouchy part of your cycle or to understand why it is you felt like crawling back under the covers this morning. Or to realize that you didn't hurt your back, you're just about to get your period. Or why you suddenly want to jump on your partner – hello ovulation. Understanding your hormonal cycle allows you to harmonize with your body's needs.

Electronic Activity Trackers: Measuring Sleep, Steps, and More

We now have available a dizzying array of fitness trackers, capable of directly measuring your heart rate 24 hours a day; calculating the number of steps you've taken and the force of impact of your running, your swimming, or your cycling workout; keeping track of the calories you've burned; and even monitoring the details of your sleep cycle. And depending on what device you choose, it may also tell time, play your music, and field your texts and emails. The prices also vary considerably, but with a little searching, it's now possible to find devices in almost any price range that will help you gather valuable measurements on your body throughout the day.

My thoughts about these seemingly miraculous devices are that absolutely no one *needs* one. You can track your fitness just fine the low-tech way. But if you love detailed feedback, or are interested in seriously improving your athletic performance, wearable technology may really work for you.

As a holistic doctor, I do feel the need to comment on the increased volume of electrical frequencies penetrating our bodies from the use of mobile phones and wearable technology. The World Health Organization's Agency for Research on Cancer issued a statement in 2011, after examining existing research on mobile phones, that mobile phones are 'possibly carcinogenic,' putting them in the same category as dry-cleaning chemicals and some pesticides, such as DDT. The issue seems to be from close proximity, as mobile-phone users with the highest frequency of use have a threefold increase in the risk of glioma, a type of brain cancer. The safe approach seems to be to keep your mobile phone away from your body whenever possible, using a headset or holding your phone away from your body. There is no research showing risks from carrying one's mobile phone on one's body, and it is worth mentioning that no credible source, including the Food and Drug Administration (FDA), the National Cancer Society, or the Centers for Disease Control and Prevention (CDC), believes there is evidence for a causal link between mobile phones and cancer. But as a physician who knows that long-term risks take a long time to surface, I am concerned about the practice of putting one's mobile phone in one's back pocket, so that it transmits through the ovaries, prostate, and testicles – cancer-prone organs that also produce our next generation. There are also a growing number of case reports of breast cancer in women in their twenties and thirties with no family history of cancer, who routinely tuck their mobile phones between their breasts.[2] We are undergoing an enormous, worldwide experiment with technology and its impact on our bodies, and we will not know the outcome for many years to come.

The issue seems to be primarily in having a 3G or 4G transmitter (a mobile phone) next to one's body. A smartwatch like the Apple Watch or the Jawbone Up uses Bluetooth and Wi-Fi, and there is currently no proof that these technologies increase cancer risk. However, some wearable technology entering the market does come with a cellular chip, and I cannot recommend these until we have better safety data. I have no problem with using wearable technology at night for a period of a week or two to track sleep cycles. But I cannot recommend wearing a sleep-tracking device or using your phone as a sleep-tracking device under your pillow on an ongoing basis. I don't even recommend having your mobile phone near your head on your nightstand. It's not necessary, and we don't yet know if it's safe. In these cases, it's better to be cautious.

With that said, if you want to explore the possibility of wearable technology to increase your ability to measure your health, the two most important things to consider when buying a device are: (1) what functions do you want and need and (2) how much do you want to spend?

If you simply want to track heart rate and steps taken, you can get away with the least-expensive trackers on the market, of which there are many. If you are a serious athlete, there are wearable devices for running and swimming that can give you detailed data about your body movement (cadence or length of stride for example) and even coach you to a better performance.

If you want an electronic activity tracker that also gives you the time and connects you to texts and emails, you may want to consider a smartwatch. These are definitely not the inexpensive option for fitness tracking, but they are pretty remarkable. If sleep monitoring is your goal, a number of devices are now available that fit under your sheet and detect motion and heat (and can also control your alarm to wake you in an advantageous time in your sleep cycle). These are probably more accurate than the wearable wristband sleep trackers, but can be disturbed by the movement of someone sleeping next to you. The wearable wristband sleep trackers are decent, and will at least give you a sense of how much you move at night and whether you are truly getting deep sleep.

Finally, if you are really one of those women who wants it all in her personal-data management, there are a few companies that are making integrated systems of activity trackers, scales with body composition, blood pressure cuffs, and sleep monitors and putting all of the data into a smartphone app that can develop a personalized coaching programme. However you choose to measure your body's wellness, from checking your own pulse to monitoring your personal data in an online programme, being aware of your own health status is an important step on the journey to being more bodywise.

Expanding Your Senses

We're all familiar with body sensations like pain, sleepiness, or being too full after Christmas lunch. But most of us, in our very busy everyday lives, spend long periods of time ignoring our bodies' sensations. We do this so that we can keep functioning. Unfortunately, many of us ignore them far too much of the time. We get carried away typing on the computer and don't register our painful neck or cramping fingers. We're in such a hurry to finish our work or care for our children that we ignore our need to eat or go to the bathroom. This ignoring has physical consequences. Too long without food can cause headaches, lightheadedness or even a sense of anxiety. Have you ever noticed how much better you feel physically when you're on holiday? Much of the improved energy and peacefulness of a holiday has to do with the ability to pay close attention to our bodies' needs for sleep, food, and movement. Becoming bodywise is about bringing that sensitivity into our everyday lives. And it all starts with being able to sense what our bodies are feeling.

When a patient comes to see me at my office with stomach pain, my first questions are always about the sensation, timing, and location of the pain. Does it hurt before or after eating (an ulcer versus gastritis)? Is it a sharp and stabbing pain (gas, obstruction, or diverticulitis) or an aching, gnawing pain (ulcer, gastritis, or intestinal inflammation)? Is it constant (intestinal inflammation) or does it come and go (gallbladder or gastritis)? Is it in your upper right abdomen (gallbladder and liver) or the lower left abdomen (ovary, diverticulitis, or intestinal inflammation)? These questions allow me to understand the language of the body and what the source of the pain might be. Being able to closely sense what your body is feeling allows you to be your own diagnostician.

If you're having trouble imagining what you might notice if you pay attention, take a look at the list of 'Body Sensations' below. How many of these can you identify in your own body? The more vocabulary we can develop for describing our sensations, the more nuanced our body wisdom can be.

Let's start with a simple body-awareness exercise. You can relax and listen to an audio version of this exercise at doctorrachel.com by clicking on *BodyWise* in the books section. You can also follow this exercise and all of the exercises in this book on our video course for *BodyWise* at RodaleU.com.

BODY SENSATIONS		
Dense	Thick	Flowing
Breathless	Fluttery	Nervous
Queasy	Expanded	Floating
Heavy	Tingly	Electric
Fluid	Numb	Wooden
Dizzy	Full	Congested
Spacey	Trembly	Twitchy
Tight	Hot	Bubbly
Achy	Wobbly	Calm
Suffocating	Buzzy	Energized
Tremulous	Constricted	Warm
Knotted	Icy	Light
Blocked	Hollow	Cold
Disconnected	Sweaty	Streaming

Source: Peter A. Levine, PhD. *Healing Trauma: A Pioneering Programme for Restoring the Wisdom of Your Body* (Sounds True: Boulder, CO), 2008, p. 50.

Exercise 3: Body Awareness

1. Close your eyes if you are able to listen to this exercise on our audio version at doctorrachel.com. For most, it is easier to focus inwardly when you are not distracted by what you see outwardly. Otherwise, it is fine to simply relax and read the exercise.
2. Sit or lie in a comfortable position.
3. Take three deep breaths. Breathe in through your nose, allowing your belly to expand, as we did in the Belly Breathing exercise on page 21.
4. Bring your awareness to each part of your body from your toes up to your head.
   - Feet and toes: Bring your awareness to the toes of your left foot. Notice whether you feel any sensation in the toes of your left foot. You might notice that simply bringing awareness to your left foot creates a sense of warmth or tingling that was not there before. Bringing your awareness to any area of your body increases blood flow and nerve activity. Now allow your awareness to spread to your right foot and toes. Simply notice any sensations that you feel, or any difference between the left and right sides.
   - Legs and buttocks: Allow your attention to move up your calves to your knees and flow into your thighs and up to your buttocks. As you move your focus through your body, note any sensations that you feel and also if there is a lack of sensation in any particular area.
   - Pelvis and belly: Notice if you feel any sensation in your pelvic area. Sensation can have a broad range, from temperature to pressure or a sense of fullness, from tingling or bubbling to actual discomfort. Discomfort has its own range of qualities from sharp pain to dull pain to throbbing or aching. Now allow your attention to wander through your belly. Are you hungry? Full? Can you sense the movement of your digestion?

If your body is telling you that you are tired or hungry or that a muscle is sore, it is fairly straightforward to know how to take care of that need. Sometimes, sensations arise and we have no idea why we are feeling what we're feeling. 'Exercise 4: Quality of Sensation' on page 32 will allow you to gather more information about your body's sensations by exploring them in detail. Understanding the specificity of your sensations allows you to begin to be the detective that uncovers the messages of your body. You can listen to a recording of this exercise at doctorrachel.com.

If you are used to tuning into the sensations of your body, these exercises may be very easy for you. If you are like most of us, and have spent

- Chest and breasts: Feel the weight of your breasts on your chest wall. Notice your rib cage and lungs expand and contract as you breathe. Does your chest feel open and expansive or closed and tight? Focus on your heart inside of your chest. Can you sense it beating? Slow or fast? Hard or soft beats?
- Back and shoulders: Bring your attention to the strong muscles of your lower back. Any pain or discomfort there? Move your awareness up your back and shoulder blades to your shoulders. Notice whether your shoulders feel easy and loose or tight and restricted.
- Arms and hands: Allow your focus to wander down your upper arms and lower arms to your hands and fingers, feeling your palms and each finger of your hands in turn. Any soreness present? Or tingling? Now return your attention back up your arms and shoulders to your neck.
- Neck and head: Feel the muscular back of your neck as it rises from your shoulders and back. Is it relaxed or tense? Feel the front of your neck as your breath passes through your trachea. Now focus your attention on the back of your head where it meets your neck and allow it to move over your cranium and through the inside of your head to your face, cheeks, and eyes. Do your eyes feel soft, wide, and relaxed or slightly tense?

5. Scan your body. Sweep your attention one more time from your feet all the way up your legs and torso out to your arms and fingers and up your neck into your face and head. Notice any parts of your body that seem to be speaking to you. Notice the particular sensations of those parts of your body.
6. Take a deep breath into that part of your body and remember the sensation. Open your eyes.

much of your life ignoring the sensations of your body, these exercises can be more challenging. I assure you that as you tune into your body's language more frequently, it will become much simpler to feel your sensations and notice the quality of those sensations in more detail.

If you find it difficult to sense what is happening within your body, don't worry. It can take some time to develop the ability to feel inside yourself again. I promise that it is absolutely possible and that it's well worth it! It can sometimes be helpful to touch the area of your body that you're focusing on, let's say your belly, with your hand. Some people feel sensation, and other people can visualize, or 'see,' sensation inside of their bodies. However your body talks to you is just fine.

Exercise 4: Quality of Sensation

1. Close your eyes and take a deep breath.
2. Focus on one area of your body in which you notice a sensation.
3. Breathe in as if you are breathing into that part of your body, and allow your awareness of that part of your body to expand.
4. What type of sensation do you feel? Is it sharp or dull? Is it tingling or effervescent? Is it a pressure or expansion?
5. What is the size of the sensation, if you can visualize it? As small as a seed or as large as a basketball, or somewhere in between?
6. How dense is the sensation? Heavy and dense like a dumbbell or light and airy like a cotton-wool ball or a balloon?
7. What temperature is the sensation? Cold, room temperature, warm, or hot?
8. What colour is the sensation? Does the sensation have no colour, one colour, or many colours?
9. Focus on the sensation and notice if its quality shifts with your attention.
10. Imagine that you are holding the sensation within the palms of your hands, and thank it for speaking to you through body language.
11. Take a deep breath, and open your eyes.

What If You Can't Feel a Specific Part of Your Body?

There are several common reasons that people will lack sensation in certain areas. If you grew up in a family or culture that had shame or disgust around sexuality, for example, you may have ignored your body's sensation from those 'shameful' parts. By focusing your attention and beginning to listen to the parts of your body that are silent, you can recover your ability to feel pleasure as well. When a child is physically abused by an adult, it is common for the child to survive that experience by reducing the painful sensations of the physical abuse and numbing the body. This prevents the intensity of both physical and emotional pain from overwhelming the child. This reaction is natural and is an important defence mechanism. However, when that child becomes an adult, the ongoing numbness prevents her from feeling the pain of the experience and being able to heal. Physical traumas, such as a car accident or an emergency surgery or a complicated childbirth, can also create such emotional and physical pain that we 'turn down the volume' of the body's language to escape the pain.

Bringing sensory awareness back to our bodies is the first step to healing the pain and shame that we have experienced. There is no part of the human body that is shameful. Our entire bodies deserve our attention and our care. If you have experienced physical abuse, sexual abuse, or rape in your past, tuning into the physical sensations of your body can be a difficult, but very important, step in a healing process. I would strongly advocate that, in addition to doing the exercises in this book, you seek support from a therapist trained in helping women recover from shame and trauma. There is a list of resources for therapists who are skilled in helping you listen to your body in Appendix B.

Learning to Feel

Now that we have learned to sense what is going on inside our bodies, we're beginning to speak the basic language of the body. Many people have trouble differentiating between 'sensing' and 'feeling,' as we often experience them in the body as one. For example, we associate the 'sensation' of bladder fullness with the feeling or interpretation, 'I have to pee.' But any woman who has had a bladder infection can tell you that you can 'sense' bladder fullness and not have to actually urinate. That sensation of bladder fullness is one of the major symptoms of a bladder infection – which means that women with bladder infections feel like they need to pee all of the time, even if they don't. And some women sense bladder fullness when they are anxious. The sensation is bladder fullness, but the actual emotion or feeling associated with it is anxiety. Separating the sensation from the feeling allows us to be more accurate in our interpretation. 'Does this bladder fullness mean that I really need to pee?' or 'Am I getting a bladder infection?' or 'Am I just anxious?' The feeling, or interpretation, can vary, depending on the circumstance.

Many sensations are related to emotional experiences. For example, most of us feel a squeezing or heaviness in the pit of our stomach when we are nervous or scared. The sensation is physical but the meaning of the sensation is emotional. It is not a sensation of hunger or gallbladder disease. It is the sensation of fear. Learning how to feel what the sensation means to us allows us a much deeper understanding of our body language. 'Sensing' the body is like understanding the body's basic vocabulary. 'Feeling' the body is like studying the body's poetry or metaphoric expression.

Mei is a hardworking accountant and mother of three that I began seeing as a patient several years ago. When I first saw Mei, she had abdominal pain and body rashes that had been diagnosed as eczema by several dermatologists. She had been prescribed topical steroid creams that helped clear the rashes temporarily, but they returned when she stopped using the steroid cream. We did a variety of testing, including evaluating her gut function and looking for food allergies and sensitivities that might be contributing to her rashes. After healing and balancing her gut environment and removing several offending foods from her diet, all of her rashes disappeared for some time. When I last saw Mei, she was doing better physically than she had in years. She was less stressed, had lost weight and was more fit, and had no stomach pain. However, she continued to have a rash around her right eye and on her right index finger only. This rash had appeared after a stressful experience with her husband's family.

Exercise 5: Body Feelings

You can find the audio version of this exercise at doctorrachel.com by clicking on BodyWise in the books section.

1. Take three deep breaths as we did in the Belly Breathing exercise, and relax into a sitting or lying position.
2. Scan your body as we did in the Body Awareness exercise, beginning with your toes and feet and moving upward to your legs, pelvis, belly, back, arms, neck, and head.
3. Focus your attention on one part of your body that seems to be talking to you. If there are several areas in which you feel sensation, choose one for which you don't have an easy explanation for the sensation.
4. Explore the quality of the sensation as we did in the Quality of Sensation exercise. What type of sensation is it? What is its size, density, temperature, or colour?
5. Imagine yourself right next to that area of sensation. One way to do this is to imagine that you are holding that sensation in the palms of your hands. Another way to imagine it is to see yourself inside a tiny spaceship that has travelled through your body to that area.
6. Ask this area of your body, 'What are you trying to tell me?' Another version of the question would be, 'What do you need to say?' Or simply, 'I'm listening.' Continue to breathe deeply into that area and be patient. You may get a verbal response in your mind. Alternately, you may see a change in your visualization of the sensation or body area, like a dream image, that speaks to you in pictures. Or a memory may arise. Or you may feel a subtle, or not-so-subtle, change in the sensation. Your job is to pay attention to whatever happens. Spend as much time as you'd like, but at least 1 minute, in this conversation with your body.
7. Thank the area of your body that you are working with, whether you have received information or not.
8. Take a deep breath, and open your eyes.

In my office, I had Mei do 'Exercise 3: Body Awareness' and 'Exercise 4: Quality of Sensation' to sense what was going on in her eye and hand. Then, I asked her to have a conversation with the rash on her right eye and her right hand. I know that this does not sound like an ordinary doctor visit, and Mei had never done exercises like these before. But when I had her feel into the sensation of her right eye and right finger and then ask those areas of her body what they were trying to tell her, here is what she heard: 'I am pointing my right finger at my in-laws and squinting my right eye and glaring at them. I'm angry because they didn't support my husband emotionally and are critical of me and of the children.'

As with all illnesses, Mei's issues had real, physiological causes: poor digestion and a dysfunctional immune system, as well as food allergies and sensitivities. But her eczema also had emotional correlates, so that a visit with her parents-in-law could produce a rash – and produce it, metaphorically, in just those areas where she is pointing the finger of blame. Mei needed safe outlets to express her anger and a constructive way to address issues in her family. Treating Mei includes all my best traditional and holistic medical approaches, but also addresses her underlying (and largely unexpressed) anger at her extended family. I encouraged Mei to find a close friend or a women's group with whom she could share her feelings. I also asked her to explore with her therapist any other situations in her early life in which she felt criticized and how those feelings could be adding to the fire of her anger. Mei is learning to listen to what her body is telling her. And those messages are not just reducing her rashes, they are helping her to create a life that she can thrive in.

When I have patients or students do this exercise, invariably some of them feel nothing or get no response. Others feel changes in the sensation, but not much else. And still others, like Mei, get very clear messages from their bodies. Mei's body spoke to her in a verbal language that she understood. This made it much easier for Mei to know what to do with the information. It is just as common to receive body language that is different from spoken language.

When you explore your body feelings, you may, for example, be shown an image or a memory of something that has happened. Remember Sofia from the Introduction (see page xiv), who had dream images of a snake biting her in the head and neck and was later diagnosed with tumours in both of those areas? It takes some good discernment and detective work to understand how these visual images are related to your health and well-being – but it is rewarding and sometimes lifesaving to do so. Spend a little time considering your experience. You may even want to write it down, draw it, or share it with someone close to you.

When you do 'Exercise 5: Body Feelings' (page 34) you may notice that the sensation you are focusing on changes. It might be more intense or disappear entirely. What this means for each individual person will vary, of course. When Kati first tried the exercise, she decided to listen to the pain in her feet, which had been hurting her for a month or so. When she focused her attention on her foot pain, the pain actually disappeared. No words or images from the pain – it just went away. And stayed away. When I spoke with her weeks later, she said, 'Yes, they still don't hurt, even after exercising, which usually makes them hurt more.' She noted that when her feet stopped hurting, she realized that the super-cute shoes she had been trying to wear (in a half-size too small) were probably not a great choice. Kati used to be a dancer; she had spent so many years in pointe shoes that she assumed that foot pain was just going to be a constant state for her. But when she actually tried the body feelings exercise, she discovered that the pain was being caused by a very specific and controllable issue – her cute-but-too-small shoes. Now, she has no foot pain *and* a great reason to go and buy a *new* pair of cute shoes – in her size. An opportunity for bodywise shoe shopping.

Finding Discernment

The BodyWise Protocol allows us to learn the language of the body. *Measure* allows us to collect data and information that inform our language. *Sense* helps us develop a vocabulary for how the body speaks. *Feel* helps us understand the metaphoric expression of the body. And *discernment* is putting measure, sense, and feel together to create a story that explains the meaning of what the body is trying to tell us. Discernment is the ability to judge well. Bodywise discernment allows us to understand what our bodies are trying to communicate to us in any given moment. Discernment is not a story that another person can tell us, because it needs to arise from our own personal experience. Other people can be great allies in discovering what might be going on, but it is really your embodied experience that makes you uniquely able to discern what your body is trying to tell you.

Discernment in Practice

Tessa is a bright, lively human relations manager who has been very successful in her career. At 32, she is now looking for a life partner and is interested in starting a family. Tessa had been dating a man who was wonderful in many ways, but their relationship always felt a bit like a struggle. Tessa had decided it was time to move in or move on, and was packing her things to move in with her boyfriend when she noticed something unusual happening. Tessa has had poison ivy, a nasty skin reaction common in the US, many times in the past, but is always able to control its spread with topical medications and careful behaviour. She already had a very small patch of poison ivy on her hand, but as she lifted her rack of clothes out of her closet to pack them, she noticed that the poison ivy was spreading from her hand all the way up her wrist and onto her arm. She thought this was odd but, as the day progressed, the poison ivy progressed as well, onto both her hands *and* arms. As she continued to pack, the poison ivy spread onto her torso and became severe in a way she was completely unused to.

In this scenario, Tessa had observational data (*measure*) – poison ivy spreading over her arms and torso in an unusual fashion. When she took a moment to check in with herself (*sense*), she had tightness and a sense of nausea in her stomach. Relating this to her feelings, she thought that the stomach discomfort was from fear about her upcoming move (*feel*). Not knowing what all of this meant, and itching uncontrollably, Tessa arranged to spend the weekend with her girlfriends rather than moving in with her boyfriend. While there, she had an opportunity to speak with her friends at length about her relationship and her concerns. She came to the painful realization that, for her own well-being, she needed to break off her relationship and that her body was demonstrating this to her in large, red welts (*discernment*). The decision was very painful but, amazingly, once the decision was made, the poison ivy began to recede from her torso and slowly from her arms as well. When I spoke with her about this, she emphasized, 'This really happened. Even my friends could see the withdrawal of the poison ivy rash once I decided not to move in with my boyfriend.'

Discerning Which Voices to Listen To

Not all of us have such visible physical signs that help us make difficult decisions, but when we listen, our bodies do try to advise us, in innumerable ways, what we should do. The process of discernment helps us to truly understand the wisdom of the body. Discernment is primarily an 'inside job,' meaning that it is something that you must work out for yourself. However, in addition to taking into account data from our bodies, we also use information from reliable sources, such as our doctors or close and trusted friends. Tessa, for example, was able to understand the poisonous aspect of her relationship, in part, from good counsel from her close friends.

An important part of gathering information from outside sources is being able to evaluate where the information is coming from and how accurate it is. It's important to know whose thoughts and opinions are truly trustworthy. This is not always an easy task. Here are some of the questions I ask when considering whether to listen to another person's opinion about my life.

1.   Do I believe that this person truly has my best interests in mind?
2.   Does this person have a personal agenda or bias, however well-intentioned, that may prevent her from seeing my best interests?
3.   Is this person competent and wise about the subject we are discussing?
4.   Do I feel relaxed and at ease with this person? Do my gut instincts tell me that she is trustworthy?

Even when your friend fulfils these criteria, her opinion is simply information to consider, just as you do other data about your well-being. You must go back to your body's wisdom – your gut instinct – to make a final decision.

When Is a Headache Just a Headache?

Some of the more challenging aspects of discernment are differentiating between when a physical symptom has meaning or when a headache is just a headache. After decades in clinical practice, I do believe that the body can speak to us metaphorically and manifest physical illness, discomfort, and pain, like Tessa's poison ivy. I also firmly believe that not all illness or pain has emotional or psychological roots. If you are mothering a snotty-nosed toddler, you are very likely to get sick. A lot. This doesn't necessarily mean something profound about your body or your relationship with your child.

However, if you are having a pattern of becoming ill every time one of your friends or family members has a cold, it could mean that your resistance is compromised. Perhaps you need more sleep, better nutrition, or a less-stressful schedule. When I had 2-year-old twin toddlers in preschool and a 6-year-old in first grade, I got sick every 2 weeks for the entire winter – including two bouts of strep throat. Most of my ills could be blamed on excessive exposure. It was certainly true that if I had had more sleep, and perhaps if I could have remembered to take vitamins and immune-boosting herbs, I may have become sick less often; at that time in my life, I could barely remember to take a shower. But the truth is, as my children got older, my exposure to infectious illnesses decreased. My sleep also increased (thank God). And now it is rare for me to become ill with a virus. My getting ill was not a metaphoric expression of my body – it was evidence that the germ theory really does work. And that I really could have done with a nap.

I want to differentiate between the process of listening to the language of your body with discernment, and the conclusion that some people draw from this process – that we are responsible for all of our own pain and illness. I want to be clear that, yes, how we think and feel, our responsiveness to our bodies' clues, and the behaviours that we choose absolutely affect our health. And ignoring the obvious cues from your body that something is wrong can manifest in more serious illness. But it is not true that we are personally responsible for the illnesses that we have. What I mean is, sometimes 'shit happens.' This was my not-so-eloquent response at a public talk to a very spiritual, healthy young woman who was diagnosed with leukaemia. The panel I was sitting on included experts on the mind-body connection and its impact on illness. The young woman at this talk was very upset by the implication that if you are ill, it's your fault, and she wanted to know if we believed that she had caused her own cancer by her thoughts or behaviours. This is a subtle distinction, but the fact that we *can* influence pain and illness with our thoughts and behaviours does not mean that we *cause* all of our pain and illness. My vegan meditation and yoga teacher patient got cancer last year. Sometimes, shit happens. Blaming illness on the person suffering (especially if that person is you) is never helpful.

If someone, including you, wants to make meaning of the illness – I need to take more time to rest or be with those that I love or eat more healthily – that is perfectly legitimate. That is not the same as 'I caused my illness by not doing those things.' We should listen to our bodies and discern the meaning of pain and illness. We must not get bogged down in the cycle of self-blame or shame about having the illness.

So, how do we tell the difference between 'shit happens' and 'my rash is telling me to break up with my boyfriend'? By using the four steps of body wisdom. Collect the data and information you need to understand your dilemma or illness. Pay attention to the sensations you feel inside your body as you go through the body awareness exercise (see page 30) and the quality of sensation exercise (see page 32). Notice what feelings arise from your awareness of those sensations. It is important to recognize that, although all four steps of body wisdom are necessary, they don't necessarily have to proceed in a particular order. For example, Sofia, whom you met in the Introduction, began to have fatigue (a heaviness in her body) and aching in her muscles (sense). She then had a dream image of a snake biting her head and neck, as well as a deeply felt emotion that something was wrong (feel), long before she was able to gather information from me as a physician, or data from blood tests and an MRI (measure). Discernment is the final step in this process, where you take all of the information gathered from outside sources, as well as your body's sensations, feelings, and intuition, and come up with a hypothesis – a story – of why you are not well and what you might need to become well.

Setting the Stage

To set the stage for the process of discernment, it is important to clear your mind and your agenda in order to truly listen to your heart and body. Some of my patients like to do this through meditation practice, sitting in silence and focusing on their breath, using belly breathing (see exercise on page 21), for example. This is akin to a mindfulness meditation practice. Mindfulness is defined by Jon Kabat-Zinn, the creator of the mindfulness meditation movement, as 'the awareness that emerges through paying attention on purpose, in the present moment, and nonjudgmentally to the unfolding of experience moment by moment.' Other patients find it helpful to go walking in nature, to go swimming, or to take a shower. What connects all of these experiences is that they are nonverbal – allowing your mind to work creatively outside of the box of verbal language. This state is also similar to what author, coach, and sociologist Martha Beck calls 'wordlessness.' Beck says this about wordlessness: '. . . it shifts consciousness out of the verbal part of the brain and into the more creative, intuitive, and sensory brain regions. Which is more powerful? Well, the verbal region processes about 40 bits of information per second. The nonverbal processes about 11 million bits per second. You do the math.'[3]

When we engage our unconscious minds, powerful messages can come forth. As we discussed previously, Mei already knew that she had eczema and that it was related to her diet and to stress. But when she took a moment to focus on what her body was telling her, it became clear that her anger at her husband's family was expressing itself through the rash of eczema on her finger and her eye. In addition to diet changes and stress reduction, she needed to focus on processing her anger to feel better. Finding a moment for mindfulness or wordlessness can be essential to unlocking the puzzle of illness or disease. When we are in that moment of wordlessness, we may have a sudden insight, connect experiences that we did not think were connected, or have a visual image that gives us a message.

I recently had a period of intense activity in my life. Wonderful opportunities were packed so tightly into my schedule that I felt less than wonderful in my body. During this phase, I had a night of stressful nightmares and jaw-clenching that led to me waking up with neck pain. When I took deep breaths and went into my body and asked the pain in my neck what it had to tell me, I received quite a tirade in response. Some of the messages were verbal, for example, 'Stop being so self-critical.' But the most helpful message was an image of my spine showing that the vertebrae were packed so tightly that the nerves coming out from between the vertebrae were being squeezed, and this was causing my neck pain.

This may be anatomically true – clenching my jaw and having muscle spasms in my neck probably *were* causing inflammation in my cervical nerve as it exited the spinal column in my neck. But what I understood from the image at a deeper level was that the spinal column that was being shown to me was a metaphor for my life. That just as the vertebrae need space between them for blood to flow and nerves to be well-supported, *I* needed space between my activities for my heart and soul to have smooth flow and to be well-supported. Listening to my body helped me to say no, even to wonderful opportunities, because the plethora of opportunities was preventing the flow of joy in my heart and soul.

Another method for honing discernment is through conscious movement. Steve Sisgold, who wrote a book called *Whole Body Intelligence*, uses a process of observing body movement in order to help his clients understand what is really holding them back from full health and vitality.[4] How we hold ourselves and how we move our bodies expresses our thoughts and beliefs, even if we're not consciously aware of them. One of the more interesting workshop exercises I have experienced asked the participants to walk across a room with shoulders hunched, chest collapsed, and head down, staring at the ground. And then to feel what emotions arise in their bodies – for me, sadness, loneliness, depression. Then walk across the room again with shoulders relaxed and back and chest open, meeting the eyes of the people you see, and smiling. This feels remarkably happy, joyful, and connected. It is true that when we feel sad, we may walk or sit in this way. But it is also true that when we make the movements consistent with sadness, we *feel* sad. The emotion creates the body posture, but the body posture also creates the emotion. Sisgold uses the observation of body posture and movement to draw out emotions and beliefs in his clients, much as trauma therapists or manual therapists trained in somato-emotional work do. Somato-emotional work focuses on how emotions impact the body and live in the tissues. Chronic body postures and tensions developed through negative emotional experiences become habitual, and the postures then re-create the negative emotion itself.

We can draw on our body intelligence through movement. Focus on an illness or dilemma that is currently happening in your life. Take a few minutes to use the BodyWise Movement exercise (see overleaf) to assist in your feeling and discernment through movement.

Exercise 6: BodyWise Movement

1. Take three deep breaths and relax into a sitting, lying, or standing position.
2. Focus your attention on an illness or dilemma, preferably one that is currently happening in your life.
3. Scan your body, beginning with your toes and feet and moving upward to your legs, pelvis, belly, back, arms, neck, and head, paying attention to what you feel in each area of your body.
4. Explore the quality of any prominent body sensations. What type of sensation is it? What is its size, density, temperature, or colour?
5. Gently allow your body to move in any way it wants to. It's common to experience shaking or trembling as a natural letting go of a previous fear or trauma. Someone who feels trapped and perhaps suffers from chest pain or shortness of breath may find herself flapping her arms and opening her chest as her body attempts to heal itself. Or, you may find yourself belly dancing or jamming to your own internal melody.
6. If it feels right, let yourself vocalize. Sing, speak, scream, growl, bird-call, or whistle. Let your voice free as your body moves. Continue to move and vocalize until your body feels complete. This may be 30 seconds, or 30 minutes. Try to pay attention to what wants to happen. When you are ready, rest in any comfortable position. Breathe deeply and relax. Allow your body to 'speak' to you in any way it wants. Saying or imagining the words 'I'm listening' can be helpful here. Listen for words, notice memories or visions, and note sensations and feelings.
7. Thank your body for speaking with you, whether you have received information or not.

How does your body's moving language influence your discernment process? Moving discernment is natural for some and more challenging for others. Sometimes, there is no verbal insight, but a transformation happens through the therapeutic effect of the movement itself. This 'release' of movement is the body's process of healing itself.

It's important to emphasize that discernment is a process of creating hypotheses. No one is perfect at discernment. We attempt to understand ourselves and our bodies to the best of our ability, but sometimes our attempts to heal ourselves are unsuccessful. Or, we think we know why we're ill and discover later that it had nothing to do with our previous 'discernment.' And because we are trying to discern our bodies' stories in lives that continue to unfold, discernment about what is true for you now could be very different from the discernment you had about the same subject area

5 years ago. Learning the language of your body is a process, much like learning any foreign language. In the beginning, you can only communicate with simple phrases, but, with time and practice, you can even appreciate metaphoric poetry in that language. Be easy with yourself in the process. Try out your hypotheses, and see if they work. Discuss them with trusted friends. And keep listening to the deep source of wisdom that is your body.

PART TWO

Overcoming Chronic Body Depletion

Whether you are barrelling ahead so fast that you don't even realize that your body is trying to communicate, or whether you hear the signals that your body is sending and choose to ignore them, chronic body depletion is your body's way of throwing up traffic cones to get you to slow the heck down. When we are pushing too hard, sleeping too little, and eating poorly, our bodies respond with a variety of symptoms. If we don't change our behaviours or our circumstances, those symptoms escalate into a predictable set of issues: chronic body depletion. The symptoms of chronic body depletion – exhaustion, chronic pain, low libido, anxiety and depression, and allergy and autoimmune disease – are very common. Whether you are experiencing one symptom acutely or all five on some level, it is always possible to lean in more closely to hear what your body has to say, and to then work with that body wisdom to heal the source of your discomfort. This part of the book can help you start listening to your own body's symptoms, understand why you have them, and find a path out of depletion and into vibrant living. At the beginning of each chapter is a quiz aimed at helping you gauge how important this particular topic is for you. You may want to concentrate on the sections that are most relevant for your health at this time. In the BodyWise 28-Day Plan at the end of the book, we'll use those quiz scores to guide your individualized plan for recovery and renewal.

CHAPTER 3

Where's the Snooze Button?
Ending Fatigue

Fatigue Quiz

1. How often do you feel tired to the bone, other than when you are ill?

1	2	3	4	5
(Never)	(Rarely)	(Sometimes)	(Usually)	(Almost always)

2. Does feeling tired keep you from doing things that you need to do (earning money, doing household work, exercising, food shopping)?

1	2	3	4	5
(Never)	(Rarely)	(Sometimes)	(Usually)	(Almost always)

3. Do you ever feel like your body is depleted of energy?

1	2	3	4	5
(Never)	(Rarely)	(Sometimes)	(Usually)	(Almost always)

4. Do your muscles ever feel like they are simply too weak to want to move?

1	2	3	4	5
(Never)	(Rarely)	(Sometimes)	(Usually)	(Almost always)

If you scored:

4–9: minimal symptoms of fatigue

10–14: moderate symptoms of fatigue

15–20: significant symptoms of fatigue

Add the numbers of your answers.
Your Fatigue score is: _____

Fatigue can be understood as tiredness, exhaustion, or lack of energy or motivation. From 'I don't want to get out of bed' to 'I can't get off the floor,' fatigue is the most common complaint that I hear from women who see me for the first time. Figuring out why most women are tired is often not that complicated. By the time I hear about their work, their relationships, their diets, their activity levels, and, most important, their sleep, we both have a very clear picture of why they're exhausted! An important part of helping my patients recover from their exhaustion is helping them to listen to what they need and to understand why they do or do not heed their own body wisdom. Helping with fatigue involves finding what it is that each woman needs to support her energy level, and examining what underlying beliefs are getting in the way of her taking action.

Melissa is a smart, committed 32-year-old mother with short brown hair and dark circles under her eyes, who came in complaining of exhaustion, anxiety, low sex drive, and weight gain. She was sleeping with her 15-month-old toddler and nursing him about five times throughout the night. Melissa worked 32 hours a week as a high-level accountant. She started work at home at 5:00 a.m. Her husband got up with their son a few hours later and cared for him until his morning nap at 10:00 a.m. She cared for him after he got up and tried to squeeze in another hour or two of work during his afternoon nap. She craved caffeine and sugar and ate ice cream every night. As is true for all of us, Melissa made decisions about diet, sleep, and work based on what she felt was most important to her and her family – not necessarily what was best for her body.

The key to understanding what was driving Melissa was finding out that when she was a child, her own mother was neglectful. I empathized with how much Melissa wanted her child to feel loved and wanted to help her understand that taking care of herself is the best gift she can give to her child. As the old saying goes, 'If Mama ain't happy, ain't *nobody* happy.' My prescription for Melissa included moving toward weaning her baby at night, thus allowing her to sleep longer, and also getting reliable childcare that she felt good about. She also saw a naturopathic doctor and an acupuncturist in my clinic who helped her with herbs and acupuncture for anxiety and sleep. These efforts helped decrease her anxiety, improve the quality of her sleep, and control her ice-cream cravings. Mostly.

Of course, there are more complex cases, where women eat well, sleep enough – perhaps too much – and yet can't even walk to the postbox. These are more serious diagnoses of chronic fatigue that require more testing and investigation to figure out the underlying causes, and we'll examine that later in the chapter. But whether fatigue is of the common variety or is representative of a more concerning medical problem, the fundamentals of restoring ourselves to health are the same: If you're tired all the time, it's difficult to enjoy your life, love the people you love well, and do your best work.

Here are all the body stresses that contribute to fatigue.

1. Lack of consistent, refreshing sleep
2. Adrenal fatigue
3. Nutritional deficiencies
4. Medical conditions: hypothyroidism, anaemia, autoimmune diseases, chronic viral infections, cancer, kidney and liver disease, diabetes, heart disease, chronic lung disease
5. Medications, drugs, and alcohol
6. Being sedentary
7. Toxic exposure

Depression and lack of meaning are also big contributors to feelings of fatigue. We'll cover them as well as the other heavy hitters like sleep, eating, and nutrition, and the importance of movement in full detail later on in the book. In this chapter, we will focus on how each of the items above specifically relates to the experience of fatigue.

Lack of Consistent, Refreshing Sleep

Good sleep is fundamental to just about everything – mood, health, intelligence, strength, creativity, ability to relate to others, sex drive – that we value in our human experience. And it is, of course, directly related to our level of energy. This does not come as a surprise to anyone, but it is amazing how often the question 'Why am I tired?' in my office comes down to not getting enough good-quality sleep. The *average* person needs 8 hours of sleep per night – meaning that half of us need *more* than 8 hours. And the number of people who actually thrive on 6 hours of sleep is very small. Between a pressured work schedule, small children, exposure to multiple screens (computer, phone, tablet, television), artificial light, putting everyone else's needs first, and *lots* of coffee – most of my patients don't sleep nearly enough. And, even if you can succeed in going to bed at a reasonable hour, anxiety and hormonal changes (especially after age 40) can make *falling* and *staying* asleep challenging. There is no substitute for getting enough sleep. No supplement or exercise regime can make up for the damaging effects of chronic sleep deprivation, and nothing will age you

> There is no substitute for getting enough sleep. No supplement or exercise regime can make up for the damaging effects of chronic sleep deprivation, and nothing will age you faster.

faster. There are wonderful strategies for helping all women to sleep well, from help going to sleep to help staying asleep in Chapter 9.

And sometimes, fatigue is a result of other conditions.

Adrenal Fatigue

Adrenal fatigue takes away your technicolour world and makes it feel black-and-white. It's hard to get out of bed in the morning or ever feel rested. Your energy is low, your motivation is low, your concentration has gone to hell, and your sex drive has disappeared completely. To really understand adrenal fatigue, you have to explore how you got so tired in the first place – from your overactive stress response.

In Chapter 2, we discussed the fight-or-flight stress response – that sympathetic nervous system activation that increases your pulse, blood pressure, and breathing rate in the face of perceived danger. Hormonally, when we enter the fight-or-flight response, our adrenal glands are activated to produce adrenaline (and noradrenaline), which causes the physiological changes of the stress response (dilated pupils, blood leaving the digestive organs and flooding the big muscles of the arms and legs, racing heart, and fast breathing). Now, adrenaline is a powerful hormone (imagine far more coffee than you should drink) and can actually cause damage to your cells from over-activation. So the body mitigates this risk by secreting cortisol – our natural steroid hormone – to limit the cellular damage wrought by too much adrenaline.

Cortisol also helps with quick energy by releasing sugar stores from the liver and increasing muscle breakdown to liberate amino acids for fuel. The acute stress response is important to our survival and, in ideal circumstances, is short-lived. The problem for humans is that with our very big brains, we are capable of extending the stress response with memories and fear of the future or dread from the past. We can also prolong the stress response by continuing to ruminate about the threat. This chronic stress response is dangerous for our health. It results in perpetually high blood sugar, loss of muscle mass, high blood pressure, lowered immune response, and disturbed sleep.

Many adults suffer adverse effects due to stress. And many GP appointments are in some way related to stress. A prolonged stress response bathes the body in excess cortisol and adrenaline, which can lead to myriad health effects, including cardiovascular disease, osteoporosis, intestinal disorders, weight gain and obesity, cancer, and anxiety and depression. Prolonged stress may be one of the risk factors that puts populations who are under threat – residents of high-crime areas, refugee populations, oppressed minorities, victims of domestic violence – at a much higher risk of illness and disease.

Our bodies are designed to maintain homeostasis – the careful balance of hormones, electrolytes, and neurotransmitters – so that we can function optimally. When a hormone, such as cortisol, is elevated for a prolonged period of time, your body attempts to bring it back into the normal range. It does this by 'down-regulating' or reducing the number of cortisol receptors, *despite* the experience of ongoing stress. We call this state adrenal fatigue. (Although at the moment, this is not commonly recognized as a condition in the UK and you might find that your GP will not endorse this. However, in the US 'holistic medical community' this is more widely recognized and it is possible to find private doctors in the UK who can do the same.) Stress, whether physical, emotional, or both, remains high, but cortisol levels drop below normal. This state is characterized by fatigue and a variety of other symptoms listed in the box below.

The symptoms of adrenal fatigue are pretty nonspecific. Someone suffering from these same symptoms could be perimenopausal, have a hypothyroid condition, or have a chronic illness, for example. This is why testing for adrenal fatigue, and other specific causes of fatigue, is so important.

Emotional Causes of Stress

- Situational stress
  - Relationship/family problems
  - Marriage
  - Divorce
  - Shifting home environment
  - Work issues
  - Financial challenges
  - Death or illness of a loved one
  - Lack of safety in one's home
  - Threat of violence
  - Racism or other bias
- Unresolved emotional stress
  - Worry
  - Anger
  - Guilt
  - Anxiety
  - Fear
  - Depression
  - Shame

Physical Causes of Stress

- Excessive exercise
- Surgery
- Medications
- Injury
- Illness and infection
- Inflammatory foods
- Exposure to environmental toxins
- Chronic or severe allergies
- Overwork and night-shift work
- Sleep deprivation
- Temperature extremes
- Chronic pain, illness, or inflammation

Symptoms of Adrenal Fatigue

- Fatigue
- Anxiety (wired and tired)
- Difficulty waking up in the morning despite good sleep
- Irritability/moodiness
- Heart palpitations
- Foggy thinking
- Weight gain
- Recurrent infections
- Poor memory
- Headaches
- Insomnia
- Hypoglycaemia (low blood sugar)
- Depression
- Lightheadedness when going from sitting to standing
- Sweets/caffeine/salt cravings
- Low sex drive

In my clinic, when I am concerned about the possibility of adrenal fatigue, I measure cortisol levels in my patients. This can be done with a blood test. However, cortisol has a natural diurnal rhythm – it is highest in the morning and gradually lowers throughout the day to be lowest before bed, when you need to rest. In order to look at the cortisol curve, it is necessary to measure it throughout the day. This is most easily done by measuring it in saliva – where it approximates the blood level of cortisol. I will often ask patients to collect samples (typically four) throughout the day to see whether their 'cortisol curve' is normal.*

The good news is that we can treat adrenal fatigue. The first order of business is to try to reduce the emotional and physical stress response. Your bodywise practice will help you listen to what your body is telling you about your life situations. What aspects of your life experience are increasing your stress response? Which of these situations can you modify? Sometimes, your health prescription may include finding a new job, leaving your abusive relationship, or getting help for physical illnesses or support for a healthy diet. And for the situations that you cannot change (your family of origin, for

* Salivary cortisol testing is not available through the NHS in the UK, but some private doctors, particularly holistic ones, can do it for you.

example), can you find ways to reduce your own stress response to these situations?

Reducing your stress response can be done with a simple belly breathing exercise (see page 21). Any form of meditation or prayer, including the moving meditations of yoga, tai chi, or qigong, can help. Gentle exercise – walking, for example – especially if it is outside in nature, is very healing for the adrenals. Getting adequate, good-quality sleep is absolutely essential.

Healthy eating goes a long way toward supporting optimal adrenal function – supplying the nutrients your body needs to combat stress and heal. 'The Adrenal Recovery Eating Plan' below is a guide to help you with this. An adrenal healing diet minimizes or excludes alcohol, caffeine, and sugar, as well emphasizing fruits, vegetables, and healthy proteins. Because of the low-blood-sugar crashes caused by inadequate cortisol levels, eating small meals that include fat and protein more frequently throughout the day works best for most women. Certain nutrients are key for adrenal functioning; eating foods with these nutrients (primarily in dark-coloured fruits and vegetables, nuts and seeds, legumes, and whole grains), or taking them as supplements, can be helpful. You'll find a list of supplements that support adrenal recovery in 'Key Nutrients for Fighting Stress' on page 55.

There are also a number of herbs that are supportive of the adrenal gland. These can be taken as supplements in capsule or tincture. A few of these, such as ashwagandha (Indian ginseng), Rhodiola, and holy basil, are pretty safe and are balancing for the adrenal glands whether you are in an acute stress response (high cortisol) or in adrenal fatigue (low cortisol). Several

The Adrenal Recovery Eating Plan

MINIMIZE

* Red meat
* Dairy
* Caffeine
* Alcohol
* Refined grains and flour
* Refined sugar
* Processed foods
* Trans fats (hydrogenated oils)

EMPHASIZE

* Foods grown, fed, and/or processed without pesticides, hormones, or antibiotics
* Fruits and veggies
* Whole grains
* Beans and legumes
* Nuts and seeds
* Good fats like olives, nuts, nut butters, and nut oils, avocados, coconut
* Cold-water fish and lean protein

other herbs can be useful, but I would strongly recommend both blood tests and a consultation with a knowledgeable practitioner experienced in treating adrenal fatigue prior to using them. Liquorice, for example, can support the cortisol levels in someone with adrenal fatigue but could exacerbate an elevated cortisol level in someone with an acute stress response, whose cortisol is already high. It can also raise blood pressure and needs to be used with caution. Ginseng is another wonderful adaptogen (balancing herb) that can support adrenal function, but there are several types of ginseng, and some can increase anxiety and blood pressure. Maca is a Peruvian root that can also beautifully support energy and mood. Again, getting a consultation from a medical doctor, naturopathic physician, acupuncturist, or chiropractor who is familiar with treating adrenal dysfunction is important.

Nutritional Deficiencies

Skipping Meals

One of the more obvious nutritional causes of fatigue is not eating *enough*. I know this sounds obvious, but it is fairly common for women to skip breakfast and eat a late lunch, effectively having an 18-hour fast without meaning to. The body needs fuel, and if you haven't eaten for an extended period of time, you can feel quite run-down. Breakfast can be simple: wholegrain toast with nut butter, an egg or two, fruit and nuts, or a smoothie with fruit, greens, and protein powder. It is also true that when you go for long periods of time without eating, you leave your body craving quick energy – sugar or fast food – and it can be more difficult to make healthy choices. Eating healthy food every 3 hours or so can be an optimal method of maintaining consistent energy throughout the day.

Foods That Make You Tired

Some foods literally *make* you tired. High-sugar foods and simple carbohydrates, like baked goods or white bagels or crisps, may spike your energy initially, which is why we crave them. Unfortunately, after the spike in your blood sugar, the blood sugar quickly drops, as simple carbohydrates do not provide sustained energy. The post-doughnut blood-sugar drop can be so severe that some women need to take a nap in order to recover their energy. Eating some healthy fat (avocados, nuts, olives) and protein with every meal helps to slow the digestion and even out blood sugar, and therefore energy, levels.

Highly processed foods, such as fast food or frozen dinners, are so laden with salt, sugar, hydrogenated oils, and other inflammatory ingredients that

Key Nutrients for Fighting Stress

- Vitamin C: 500 milligrams, one to two times daily
- Vitamin B$_6$ as pyridoxal-5-phosphate: 50 to 100 milligrams daily
- Vitamin B$_5$ as pantothenic acid: 500 milligrams, one to two times daily
- Biotin: 2.5 to 5 milligrams daily
- Magnesium citrate: 200 to 800 milligrams daily
- Zinc picolinate: 15 to 30 milligrams daily

they are literally toxic for the body. They raise your inflammatory markers and create a metabolic mess that your body then needs to clean up. The process of detoxification and combating inflammation takes energy, which is why most of us don't feel particularly energetic after our pizza delivery.

Surprisingly, caffeine can make you tired. There is no doubt that caffeine is a stimulant and that drinking caffeine in any form – tea, coffee, fizzy drinks, yerba mate (a South American herb), or energy drinks – will typically increase your concentration and energy for a period of time. Caffeine allows you to borrow from your future energy reserves for the needs of the present moment. Sometimes, this is understandable. As a previous medical resident and a mother of twins, I have definitely used caffeine to survive from time to time! But when you are exhausted – from chronic sleep deprivation, adrenal fatigue, or illness – borrowing from future energy reserves can be devastating, because there is very little energy in reserve! Although it sounds strange, caffeine is a reasonable strategy when you are actually well-rested and your energy reserves are full. If you are ill, drinking caffeine will further drain an already-compromised system and further exacerbate your ongoing fatigue. Remember, caffeine doesn't 'give' you energy, it borrows from your future energy reserves, and thus is a drain on the body. If your body cannot handle a further energy drain because of sleep deprivation or illness, caffeine can make you more tired. Listen to your body and respect your own boundaries with regard to caffeine intake. And if you are going to indulge, don't do it in toxic forms, such as cola or energy drinks. Stick to a traditional form of caffeine with other antioxidant, even disease-fighting, benefits, such as tea, coffee, or yerba mate.

Remember, caffeine doesn't 'give' you energy, it borrows from your future energy reserves, and thus is a drain on the body.

Nutrient Deficiencies That Make You Tired

A woman can have a nutritional deficiency from a poor diet that lacks the necessary nutrients, and this can be another cause of fatigue. The most common missing pieces of a nutritious diet are fruits and vegetables. And even 'healthy' diets that are restrictive in some way can be missing important nutrients. For example, a vegan diet, with no animal products, is deficient in vitamin B_{12} and the essential fatty acid DHA. A vegetarian diet that doesn't emphasize sufficient greens and beans can be deficient in iron. And a Paleo diet (without whole grains or legumes) can lack important B vitamins. Eating carefully and taking supplements to make up for missing nutrients is important if you are following a restricted diet. All vegans in my practice are on B_{12} and a DHA supplement. Most DHA supplements are derived from fish, but algae forms of DHA are also available.

Another source of nutrient deficiencies, despite a good diet, is the inability to absorb food. If you don't chew well, you don't absorb well. If you have low stomach acid (from age or from antacid medications), it impairs vitamin B_{12} and magnesium absorption. If your digestive enzymes are lacking, your protein, fat, carbohydrate, or vitamin absorption is impaired. And if you have intestinal disorders, such as coeliac disease, Crohn's disease, intestinal infections, or even bacterial overgrowth of the small or large intestine, nutrient absorption can be affected. A lack of nutrients causes fatigue because your body doesn't have the fuel (fats, carbohydrates, or protein) or the cofactors (vitamins) to produce energy inside your cells.

Strange as it may seem, you can have stellar nutrient intake and absorption and still need additional vitamins to function optimally. This is because each of us is genetically unique and processes and utilizes nutrients differently. For example, it is not uncommon for my patients to have genetic deficiencies in their abilities to use the B vitamin folic acid, and to need not only much more than the average person but also particular forms of B vitamins to function optimally (i.e., like the methylated forms: methylcobalamine and methyl folic acid).

The most common vitamin and mineral deficiencies that we find today are low levels of iron; vitamin B_{12}, folic acid, and the other B vitamins; and magnesium.

Iron

Iron is necessary for the formation of red blood cells, which carry oxygen to all the cells in your body. A lack of iron causes anaemia – too few red blood cells – and a number of symptoms, including fatigue, shortness of breath with exercise, pale skin, and thin, sparse hair. Iron is present in iron-fortified cereals, all meat, seafood, beans (especially white beans, chickpeas, and kidney beans), lentils, and leafy greens like spinach.

The most common cause of anaemia in women between menarche and menopause is blood loss from heavy or prolonged periods or the demands of pregnancy and childbirth. If you consume enough iron-rich foods or take an iron supplement, you can usually keep up with the demand for iron and avoid becoming anaemic. However, when periods are extremely heavy, additional efforts are necessary to reduce the amount of blood flow and help your body maintain its energy.

For a young woman, this might involve using a birth-control pill, ring, or patch – all of which reduce menstrual bleeding and pain. Unless there is a strong family history of breast cancer or blood clots, or a known genetic tendency toward either one of these, or other contraindications, birth control is a fairly safe treatment for extremely heavy periods, particularly when actual birth control is also desired.

Another option for heavy bleeding, from a holistic medicine perspective, is the use of natural progesterone – by which I mean progesterone that is the same chemical compound that your body makes, also known as bioidentical progesterone. Unlike the progestins (known in the UK as progestogen, or synthetic progesterone) used in prescription hormonal birth control, natural progesterone is much less likely to cause depression and vaginal dryness. In fact, in the perimenopausal time frame (the 10 years before menopause), replacing progesterone in the 2 weeks prior to menstruation, either by cream or by capsule, can reduce heavy bleeding, reduce PMS symptoms, and help with sleep. One of my perimenopausal friends calls her progesterone her 'precious' because she feels so much better when she takes it. Did I mention that natural progesterone also affects the GABA receptor and helps women feel calm and sleep deeply? As I said before, your body can have any reaction to anything, so keep in mind that despite the good fortune many of my patients have on natural progesterone, some of my patients feel like the wicked witch on *any* form of progesterone. Pay attention to what *your* body feels in reaction to any added hormones.

And if you are wanting to avoid hormones altogether, taking a herb, such as vitex (also known as chasteberry or agnus castus), which naturally boosts progesterone, or one of many herbs that reduces bleeding can also be helpful. One of my favourite recommendations for heavy, painful, and irregular periods is traditional Chinese medicine herbs and acupuncture, which are sometimes miraculously effective.

The best iron supplement to take is the one that your body responds to well. Some can cause constipation, but other forms (especially those combined with herbs and often in liquid form) are better tolerated. It's good to experiment to see which form of supplemental iron works best in your body.

B Vitamins

After vitamin-D deficiency, B-vitamin deficiencies are the most common vitamin deficiency I see in my clinic – particularly in women, and particularly in women with fatigue. Vitamin B_{12} is found primarily in animal foods in the diet (though vegan-sourced B_{12} supplements are also available). Good sources include shellfish, red meat, poultry, fish, eggs, and dairy products. It is also possible to get B_{12} from fortified nut and soy milks and cereals. B_{12} is important in energy production, red blood cell synthesis, and maintaining DNA , RNA, and nerve cells. Low B_{12} levels can cause a wide range of symptoms, including fatigue, numbness and tingling of the hands and feet, difficulty with balance, anaemia, memory issues, and weakness. I have a handful of patients every year who have extraordinary improvements in energy and mood – just by adding a B-vitamin supplement!

The B vitamin folic acid is important for energy production and healthy DNA, as well as red blood cell production. Folic acid is an important B vitamin that is essential to reducing birth defects in pregnant women, which is why there are high doses in prenatal vitamins. It is routinely added to processed grain products, such as bread or cereal, to be sure that women get enough of it so their babies are healthy. Adequate folic acid also protects you from cancer, impaired immunity, and heart disease. Good sources of folic acid are fortified grains, green vegetables, and beans and legumes. Low folic acid can result from reduced intake, but in the United States, it is more commonly poorly absorbed as a side effect of excessive alcohol intake, acid-blocking medications (omeprazole, pantoprazole, ranitidine, cimetidine, etc.), SSRI antidepressants (fluoxetine, citalopram, escitalopram, paroxetine, sertraline, etc.), NSAIDs (nonsteroidal anti-inflammatory drugs – think ibuprofen or naproxen), some diuretics, anticonvulsants, and antibiotics. This is quite a long list of medications, and it should be noted that acid-blocking medications, SSRI antidepressants, and NSAIDs are some of the most commonly prescribed medications on the market! Acid-blocking medications should not, except in very specific clinical situations, be used on an ongoing basis. They cause nutritional compromise as well as increase the risk of pneumonia and intestinal infections.

Vitamins B_1 (thiamin), B_2 (riboflavin), B_3 (niacin), B_5 (pantothenic acid), B_6, and biotin are also essential. Lacking even one of the B vitamins can impair your body's ability to turn protein, fats, and carbohydrates into energy. We can find B vitamins in whole grains, milk, cheese, eggs, poultry, organ meats, fish, lentils, and brewer's yeast. In fact, nutritional yeast, a savoury yellow powdered condiment that can be great on salads, eggs, and popcorn, has the highest concentration of all the B vitamins (other than B_{12}, which is found only in animal products). I often recommend it to women who need B vitamins but cannot tolerate taking a B-vitamin supplement. All forms of oral contraceptives and hormone-replacement therapy can reduce the levels of B_1, B_2, and B_3, as can heavy alcohol use and diuretics. I recommend that all of my patients with fatigue and all of my patients on hormonal birth control take a B-complex supplement or good multivitamin that contains adequate B vitamins.

As discussed above, if you have genetic characteristics that impair your methylation process (defects in your MTHFR, COMT, or other methylating genes), you will want to find a B supplement that includes not just folic acid and B_{12}, but methyl folic acid or methyl B_{12} (methylcobalamin). This genetic testing can be ordered by your practitioner at almost any lab, or you can actually order genetic testing online. As with any testing, be sure before you order that finding out your own genetic code is to your physical and psychological benefit. Not all information is helpful, and if you know that genetic information will increase your stress, it may be best not to find out! (In most cases, this genetic testing will not be covered by the NHS.) Alternately, you can simply try one of the B-vitamin supplements with methylated forms of folic acid or B_{12} and see how your body responds.

Magnesium

Magnesium is an essential mineral and is involved in more than 300 metabolic reactions in the body. It is a cofactor in the energy production cycle, important in bone production, and essential to nerve and muscle conduction and cell signalling. Low magnesium levels lead to fatigue, muscle weakness or spasm, constipation, depression, high blood pressure, low calcium and potassium levels, and heart arrhythmias. We get magnesium from dark leafy greens, oatmeal, buckwheat, whole grains, milk, nuts and seeds, beans, and, happily, chocolate. Causes of low magnesium include excessive alcohol use, diuretics, diabetes, and kidney disorders. Unfortunately, as many as 23 per cent of US adults have low magnesium levels.[1] And low magnesium levels have been linked to a persistent and debilitating type of fatigue, chronic fatigue syndrome.[2, 3] Magnesium is easy to supplement and comes in many forms, some of which are better for softening the stools, if needed (citrate, oxide, chloride), and others that are better absorbed for fatigue or muscle spasm (aspartate complexes seem to be particularly good for fatigue, and glycinate is also well-absorbed).

Medical Conditions That Cause Fatigue

An exhaustive discussion of all illnesses that can cause fatigue would be beyond the scope of this book and beyond your patience as a reader! However, I want you to be able to be bodywise in understanding what conditions might be worth testing for, to be sure that they are not contributing to your being tired. Let's start with hypothyroidism, as it is probably the most commonly undiagnosed medical condition that causes fatigue.

*Hypo*thyroidism means *low* thyroid function. *Hyper*thyroidism is *elevated* thyroid function and generally does not cause fatigue. It makes people 'hyper' and energetic. Thyroid hormone is essential to normal levels of energy, as it stimulates metabolism and increases the body's cellular energy production. People with low thyroid function (hypothyroidism) are tired. People with high thyroid function (hyperthyroidism) are usually overly energetic and can't sleep.

Clinicians measure thyroid function primarily based on the thyroid-stimulating hormone (TSH) level. Most labs consider a TSH up to 4.5 mU/L within the normal range. Many holistic practitioners and many endocrinologists feel that the TSH is really normal when it is less than 4. If your TSH has been sitting in the higher range of normal, you may very well be in the early stage of hypothyroidism and may benefit from thyroid support or treatment. Be sure that your health-care provider checks your thyroid status in your evaluation for fatigue, including a TSH, free T4, and free T3. Not all practitioners test free T3 and free T4, but fatigued patients with borderline thyroid function and a low free T3 (active thyroid hormone) often benefit from replacement with T3 (liothyronine), available by prescription.

Infections of all kinds can cause fatigue, from a bacterial skin infection to pneumonia to chickenpox. You'll be familiar with this, as even the common cold makes you much more tired than usual. Your body is busy using its resources to fight the infection and doesn't have leftover energy for you

Medical Conditions That Cause Fatigue

Hypothyroidism	Autoimmune diseases (rheumatoid arthritis, lupus, coeliac disease, pernicious anaemia, inflammatory bowel disease, etc.)	Kidney disease
Anaemia		Liver disease
Chronic viral infections		Heart disease
Cancer		Chronic lung disease
Diabetes		

to, say, run 10 miles. All acute infections cause fatigue for the period of the infection, usually days to a month, if you are healthy. But some infections can cause fatigue that persists for much longer. When exhaustion is easily explained by sleep deprivation or other causes, there is no need to test for infectious causes of fatigue. However, in a patient with prolonged fatigue, longer than a month, who does not have any of the other causes of fatigue, I do selectively test for infections.

For example, Chantal is a 28-year-old, previously healthy, dental hygienist who came to see me for the first time with complaints of fatigue. She had 'never been tired like this before,' and it had all started with a 'cold,' with body aches and sore throat. No matter how much she slept, she couldn't seem to get rested and was having to miss work, putting her job at risk. Her lab testing showed her to be suffering from mononucleosis caused by the Epstein-Barr virus. The treatment for this is supportive: rest, immune-enhancing herbs, and perhaps acupuncture or Chinese medical treatment. But the recovery can be long, between 1 and 6 months, and knowing her diagnosis allowed Chantal to take sick leave and resume work part-time when she was feeling better. Most of the other infectious causes of prolonged fatigue *can* be medically treated, and they are worth looking for if there has been suspected exposure or there are specific symptoms that point toward infectious causes. Seeing your doctor for guidance around diagnosis and testing is essential.

Infectious Causes of Prolonged Fatigue

- Viruses that cause mononucleosis syndrome
  - Epstein-Barr virus (EBV)
  - Cytomegalovirus (CMV)
- Viral liver infections
  - Hepatitis A, B, or C
- Intestinal parasites
- Tuberculosis
- HIV infection
- Endocarditis (bacterial infection of a heart valve)
- Lyme disease
- Herpes virus (HHV)
- Undiagnosed bacterial or fungal infections (sinusitis, pneumonia, tonsillitis, or abscesses)

Fatigue is a common complaint in my patients with severe allergies and autoimmune disease. When the immune system is constantly in reaction, as it is in autoimmune disease and allergy, your body feels as if it has a constant state of the flu – tired, achy, and with foggy thinking. Testing for autoimmune diseases and allergies is discussed in detail in Chapter 7, and if you have other symptoms of these, such as joint pain and inflammation, blood in your stools, unexplained rashes, or ongoing sneezing and congestion, you may want to pursue additional testing to look for autoimmune disease or define allergies.

Liver, kidney, heart, and lung disease, diabetes, and cancer can all have fatigue as one of their presenting symptoms. The good news is that routine cancer screening – physical examinations, cervical smears, mammograms, and routine lab tests (complete blood count, comprehensive metabolic panel, and urinalysis) – can find most of these conditions before they are dangerous for you. This is why seeing your doctor regularly for routine check-ups and screening is so important.

Regardless of the medical issues that you may have, optimizing your sleep, lowering your stress levels, and improving your nutrition will be fundamental for supporting your energy in *any* chronic illness. Remember that these three fundamentals will enhance your healing capacity and your immune function, no matter what diagnosis you may have.

Medications, Drugs, and Alcohol

As a holistic physician, one of the first questions I ask myself when my patients come in with fatigue is, 'Are we causing it?' Fatigue is a side effect of an amazing array of commonly used medications. (See the table on pages 64 to 65.) And because each of us is biochemically individual, a medication that doesn't typically cause fatigue in most people can cause fatigue in you.

The majority of my patients do *not* actually feel tired on their blood pressure medications or antidepressants, for example, but some do, and it's important to know if you are one of them. Please do not stop any medications without consulting your doctor, as some medications, including antidepressants, can have severe withdrawal symptoms. If your medication is causing fatigue, it is sometimes possible to switch to a medication with fewer fatigue side effects. Some blood pressure medications, for example, do not typically cause fatigue. It's certainly worth asking your health-care provider if there are other options for you.

In some cases, one of your medications may cause fatigue but be absolutely necessary for your health. This is the case for cancer medications, some medications for autoimmune disease, or blood pressure medication in someone with severe coronary artery disease. When you need to stay on your medication, there may be options for improving your energy despite the medication. Some medications affect nutritional parameters, for example, which can be overcome with supplementation.

Almost every commonly abused drug, including alcohol and marijuana, can cause fatigue. If you are using marijuana more than once a week, drinking more than seven drinks a week (one drink being a 175ml glass of wine, a 350ml beer, or a 45ml shot of spirits), or using any other drugs, these habits are very likely to be contributing to your fatigue. You may want to get support in how to reduce or eliminate your use of substances in order to support your overall health and energy level.

Being Sedentary

Okay, when you're exhausted, you don't want to move, right? Who wants to get off the couch when her body feels tired all the time? But the ironic truth is that the less you move, the more tired you are, with only a few exceptions. Women with chronic fatigue do, in fact, get *more* tired when they do too much. And women with chronic illnesses or adrenal fatigue can tire themselves out with too much activity as well. But with those exceptions, mild forms of activity – walking, yoga, water aerobics, or riding an exercise bike – all *increase* energy levels in most women with fatigue. One of the first things I try to get my exhausted patients to do is to find some form of movement that feels good to their bodies – even if it's just walking around the block. Getting outside has an extremely positive effect on stress and lowering cortisol and is vital in someone who is fatigued, even with adrenal fatigue. Find an activity that you enjoy, and do it regularly. You can find more guidance and assistance in Chapter 10.

Toxic Exposures

Some 50,000 chemicals have been introduced into our environment since 1950. Only a small percentage of these have been tested for safety in humans. We are just beginning to see the long-term impact of our multiple exposures. And in addition to chemicals that are foreign to our physiology, there are natural substances, such as heavy metals (mercury, aluminum, lead, etc.) that we have concentrated in our environment with modern industrial practices that can harm our physiology and nervous systems. Often, the result of the toxic exposures includes hormone disruption, nerve and brain dysfunction, and, of course, fatigue.

Most of us are able to handle the toxins to which we are exposed, but

Medications That May Cause Fatigue

- Antihistamines
  - Chlorpheniramine, promethazine, hydroxyzine, and cetirizine
- Cough and cold medicines
  - Night Nurse and others containing alcohol or antihistamines
- Blood pressure medications
  - Beta-blockers (such as propranolol, metoprolol, atenolol, nebivolol, nadolol and others)
  - Calcium channel blockers (amlodipine, nifedipine, diltiazem, verapamil, and others)
  - Alpha-blockers (prazosin, doxazosin, terazosin, and others)
  - Clonidine
- Cancer treatments
- Narcotic pain medications
  - Codeine, hydrocodone, oxycodone, methadone, and morphine
  - Hydromorphone
  - Pethidine
  - Fentanyl
  - Tramadol
- Antidepressants
  - Mirtazapine
  - Tricyclic antidepressants (amitriptyline, nortriptyline, imipramine, and others)
  - Monoamine oxidase inhibitors (selegiline and others)

when we are vulnerable – ill, nutritionally depleted, immunosuppressed, under stress – we are more susceptible to their negative impact. None of us can avoid toxins entirely, but it is possible to lessen our exposure. It is also the case that a healthy diet, with nutrients that support our liver detoxification, can help our bodies sequester and 'disarm' the toxins we're exposed to. If you suspect that you may have been exposed to specific toxins, such as mercury (in thermometers, large fish, 'silver' dental fillings) or lead (old paint, soldering – including in pipes in old homes), you may want to request a private test from a complementary therapist. It is also smart to avoid further exposures as much as possible. The list on page 66 can help you start this process as part of your BodyWise 28-Day Plan at the end of the book.

- Serotonin and norepinephrine reuptake inhibitors (SNRIs) (venlafaxine, desvenlafaxine, duloxetine, milnacipran, and levomilnacipran)
- Selective serotonin reuptake inhibitors (SSRIs) (fluoxetine, paroxetine, sertraline, citalopram, fluvoxamine, and escitalopram) Note: It is more unusual to have fatigue as a long-term side effect from SSRIs.
- Anti-anxiety medications
  - Benzodiazepines (alprazolam, lorazepam, clonazepam, temazepam, diazepam, and others)
  - Buspirone
- Antipsychotics and mood stabilizers
  - Aripiprazole, risperidone, olanzapine, and haloperidol
- Autoimmune disease medications
  - Methotrexate
  - Biologic medications (tocilizumab, certolizumab, etanercept, adalimumab, canakinumab, abatacept, infliximab, rituximab, and golimumab)
  - Hydroxychloroquine
  - Cyclosporine
  - Azathioprine
- Commonly abused drugs that cause fatigue
  - Alcohol
  - Prescription narcotics or anti-anxiety medications
  - Heroin
  - Marijuana
  - Barbiturates

Chronic Fatigue Syndrome

Chronic fatigue syndrome (CFS), also known as Myalgic Encephalomyelitis (ME), is a much more severe and debilitating form of fatigue than most of us experience. It is called a syndrome in the medical literature because we recognize the cluster of symptoms that defines the disease, but do not, as yet, thoroughly understand what causes it. It is a frustrating disease as accurate diagnosis and effective treatment can sometimes be difficult to find. And because there are no obvious external signs of illness, women suffering from ME are often accused of malingering by people around them – that is, pretending to be ill when they aren't. ME is primarily a female disease, with 60 to 80 per cent of cases occurring in women. Also, chronic fatigue strikes

Environmental Toxins to Avoid

- Household exposures
  - Teflon (polytetrafluoroethylene) nonstick pans
  - Chemical pesticides for home and garden
  - Toxic housecleaning agents (see ewg.org/guides/cleaners)
  - Lead-based paint dust
  - Mercury-containing thermometers
  - Mercury and lead in metalwork and soldering
  - Traditional paints and finishes and paint strippers
  - PVC (vinyl) products
  - Fire retardants in furniture, linens, and sleepwear
- Personal product ingredients (see ewg.org/skindeep and safecosmetics.org for more information)
  - Fragrance (both irritating and can contain hidden toxic ingredients)
  - Parabens
  - Diethyl phthalate
  - PEG/ceteareth/polyethylene
  - Triethanolamine
  - Iodopropynyl butylcarbamate
  - Retinyl palmitate, retinyl acetate, retinoic acid, and retinol in daytime products
  - Hydroquinone (a skin lightener)
  - Coal tars
  - Sunscreens with retinyl palmitate or oxybenzone (avoid aerosol spray and powder sunscreens)
  - Nail polish with formaldehyde, formalin, toluene, and dibutyl phthalate.
  - Dark, permanent hair dyes (may contain coal tars)
- Food
  - Fish that contains high levels of mercury (especially king mackerel, marlin, orange roughy, shark, swordfish, tilefish, ahi tuna, and bigeye tuna). If the whole fish fits on your plate, mercury is probably not a problem. (See nrdc.org/stories/smart-seafood-buying-guide and seafoodwatch.org.)
  - Plastic bottles made of polycarbonate #7 (which contains bisphenol A [BPA]) and cans lined with plastic containing BPA (see list of cans with BPA linings at ewg.org/research/bpa-canned-food)
  - Anything heated in plastic (including frozen food containers), even if it is labelled 'microwave-safe'

women who are often fully functional prior to diagnosis, and is thus devastating to self-esteem. Chronic fatigue is defined in the UK by NICE (National Institute for Healthcare Excellence) as significant fatigue symptoms for 4 months in an adult and 3 months in a child or adolescent.[4]

Chronic fatigue is often started by an illness that is viral in character, either a flulike illness or a gastrointestinal illness, and one of the possible causes is infection. There seem to be characteristics of both immune dysfunction and adrenal dysfunction in chronic fatigue patients. Sleep disruption is customary, and almost all chronic fatigue patients need a lot of sleep – and don't feel refreshed by the sleep they get.

As a holistic doctor, I literally consider every possible cause of fatigue that we have discussed in this chapter with each of my chronic fatigue patients. All of these issues need to be addressed and supported. I also do more extensive testing, which you could discuss with a holistic or naturopathic doctor, looking at mitochondrial energy production and cellular need

NHS Diagnostic Criteria for CFS/ME

Chronic fatigue syndrome (CFS) causes persistent fatigue (exhaustion) that affects everyday life and doesn't go away with sleep or rest. Most cases of CFS are mild or moderate, but up to one in four people with CFS have severe symptoms. These are defined as follows:

- mild – you're able to care for yourself, but may need days off work to rest
- moderate – you may have reduced mobility, and your symptoms can vary; you may also have disturbed sleep patterns and need to sleep in the afternoon
- severe – you're able to carry out minimal daily tasks, such as brushing your teeth, but have significantly reduced mobility, and may also have difficulty concentrating

The following tests should usually be done:

- urinalysis for protein, blood and glucose; urea and electrolytes
- full blood count
- liver function; thyroid function
- erythrocyte sedimentation rate or plasma viscosity
- C-reactive protein; random blood glucose
- serum creatinine; blood screening for gluten sensitivity
- serum calcium; creatine kinase

For more information, go to www.nhs.uk/conditions/chronic-fatigue-syndrome/Pages/Introduction.aspx.

Health Workup for Fatigue

- Adrenal fatigue – If you suspect you have adrenal fatigue, you should visit your GP as your first port of call, and they can carry out tests for general fatigue, although they are unlikely to diagnose adrenal fatigue as a condition. A holistic or naturopathic doctor can order salivary testing to look at your cortisol curve.
- Nutrient deficiencies – most of these can be measured with standard testing.
  1. Iron – To assess your iron status, have your physician order:
     - a complete blood count, assessing for anaemia
     - a serum iron and iron binding level
     - and a ferritin level (which is a measure of your iron storage)
  2. B_{12} – a serum B_{12} is a fairly accurate measure of deficiency. Keep in mind that the 'normal' range is 200 to 1,200 pg/ml, but a fair number of women are deficient between 200 and 400 pg/ml. If your results are in this low range, you may want to get a serum methylmalonic acid test, which is a more accurate test for B_{12} deficiency.
  3. Folic acid – Serum folic acid is a simple blood test. Note that it may be normal in a person with genetic issues with methylation (MTHFR, COMT), who would benefit from methyl folic acid.
  4. Other B vitamins (B_1, B_2, B_3, B_5, B_6) can be measured in the serum as well, though it is possible to still have an increased need for one of the B vitamins, even if the serum level is normal.
  5. Magnesium – Have your physician order a red blood cell magnesium test, which is a better measurement than a serum magnesium as it measures magnesium within the cell.
- Medical conditions
  1. Hypothyroidism – Have your physician order a TSH, free T4, and free T3. Remember that the TSH is not normal if it is close to or above

for nutrients. Although the treatment for ME can be complex, scientific understanding is in a better place than it's been in decades and almost all of my patients improve with treatment.

Ending Fatigue

Fatigue can be a debilitating, frustrating, and discouraging symptom of chronic body depletion, but do not lose heart: It will not last forever if you begin to pay attention and root out the causes of fatigue in your lifestyle and body. Use the resources at your disposal – find doctors and medical profes-

4 mU/L, and that you may have early hypothyroidism. If your blood tests are abnormal, have your physician check your TPO antibodies to see if you are having an autoimmune reaction, known as Hashimoto's disease (information about this in Chapter 7).

2. Anaemia – Have your physician order a complete blood count (CBC) to start. Other tests, such as a ferritin level, which reflects the body's iron stores, or a vitamin B_{12} or folic acid level may also be appropriate.

3. Chronic diseases – In addition to a CBC, I would recommend a comprehensive metabolic panel as an initial workup for all patients with fatigue, as it gives us information on blood sugar and diabetes and kidney and liver function.

4. Infectious diseases – If no other obvious causes are found, the fatigue is prolonged, and specific symptoms suggest infection, discuss testing for infectious causes with your doctor.

● Chronic fatigue

1. All tests above are relevant.

2. Consider measuring levels of oestrogen, progesterone, testosterone, and DHEA in the blood, as abnormal hormone production can characterize chronic fatigue and worsens the symptoms.

3. Consider in-depth nutritional testing, including urinary organic acids and amino acids, as well as comprehensive stool testing to evaluate digestive ability, inflammation, and appropriate bacterial populations. This will probably need to be done with an integrative practitioner (see resources in Appendix B).

4. Discuss appropriate supplementation with your provider.

sionals who can help you, open yourself up to trying new approaches, and listen closely to how your body responds to your efforts. In almost all cases, I have been able to help my fatigued patients get substantial, if not complete, relief of their symptoms by using all of the tools discussed above. Remember that no matter what is causing your fatigue, it will probably take some time and some experimentation for your energy levels to return to normal. But with patience, you can again have the energy to have the life you love. See the guide to tests (above) that you may want to discuss with your health-care provider.

CHAPTER 4

When It Doesn't Hurt So Good: Ending Chronic Pain

Chronic Pain Quiz

1. Does some part of your body hurt consistently every day?

1	2	3	4	5
(Never)	(Rarely)	(Sometimes)	(Usually)	(Almost always)

2. Does body pain keep you from doing things that you need to do, such as work or caregiving?

1	2	3	4	5
(Never)	(Rarely)	(Sometimes)	(Usually)	(Almost always)

3. Does body pain keep you from doing things that you want to do?

1	2	3	4	5
(Never)	(Rarely)	(Sometimes)	(Usually)	(Almost always)

4. Does body pain affect your mood or mental state?

1	2	3	4	5
(Never)	(Rarely)	(Sometimes)	(Usually)	(Almost always)

Add the numbers of your answers.
Your Chronic Pain score is: _____

If you scored:

4–9: minimal impact of chronic pain

10–15: moderate impact of chronic pain

16–20: significant impact of chronic pain

Pain and injury are the most common reasons that people visit the doctor, but in this chapter, I am not referring to an ankle sprain or twisted knee. I am talking about *chronic* sources of pain: the back or neck pain that never resolves, painful arthritis, recurrent headaches, nerve pain, fibromyalgia (a syndrome of persistent body aches), or chronic pelvic pain, to name a few of the most common. Studies show that 46 per cent of people in the United States suffer from some form of chronic pain,[1] and back pain is the leading cause of disability worldwide.[2] Acute pain is your body trying to signal to you that something is wrong. Anyone who has touched a hot stove understands that the pain of the burn is your body trying to save its skin – literally. Chronic pain is also trying to tell us something – it's just not always as clear as, 'Stop touching hot stoves!'

Understanding the experiences that exacerbate your pain, or alleviate it – and in many cases this means tuning into your body wisdom again – is vital to staying active and happy. Everyone experiences pain at one time or another, but what is it that predisposes someone to have pain that becomes a chronic problem? Certainly, some severe injuries are more likely to result in chronic pain, but it is interesting that the anatomy of the injury itself doesn't usually differentiate who gets chronic pain and who doesn't. For example, I examine many patients who I think have neck pain from nerve impingement – or, literally, a squashing of a nerve as it exits the spinal column in the neck. Yet, I don't initially order an MRI to see what is happening anatomically in the neck unless the patient has weakness or paralysis. This is because in the large majority of cases, *the degree of nerve impingement does not predict the extent of the pain.* That's right. A patient with what looks on a scan like terrible arthritis and severe nerve impingement in the neck can have less pain than someone with only slight impingement. There is something else going on with pain and sensitivity other than just anatomy. And this is even more the case with conditions such as migraines, arthritis, fibromyalgia, or pelvic pain.

Emerging research shows that structural changes in the brain make chronic pain more likely in certain individuals than in others. The following factors also make someone more likely to suffer pain chronically.[3]

- Being female (really)
- Work that requires prolonged standing, sitting, or lifting
- Smoking, alcoholism, or drug use
- Coming from a family with chronic-pain issues
- A lack of physical fitness
- Anxiety and depression

- Job stress and dissatisfaction with work
- A history of psychological, physical, or sexual abuse
- Experiencing a lack of meaning or purpose in life

An initial injury or even one's genetics – risks we can't change – actually has a very small influence in the development of chronic pain. However, a bodywise woman can change the life behaviours that increase her pain risk and give herself a greater chance of finding a life with less or no pain.

Samantha came to see me as a wise, deeply spiritual, 54-year-old woman with such severe, constant migraine headaches that she was mostly bed-bound for a year. Because she was also, at the time, a devoted mum of an active 18-year-old boy and 12-year-old girl, this was particularly difficult for her and her family. Samantha has a presence, with her riotous red hair and quick wit, and she was used to being the mum and friend that all her loved ones depended on. Now, she was in severe and constant pain and felt helpless. Her other doctors prescribed migraine medication and opioids, which she became dependent on, but nothing really helped. When I saw Samantha, I was touched by the spiritual maturity and insight in someone who was physically suffering so much that she had to see me in a dark room, lying down.

We worked with Samantha's body intelligence to guide the direction of treatment, since intuition was a well-developed skill of hers. She told me that the opioids weren't helping and that she knew she needed to stop them. I helped her wean off of them slowly with no worsening in her pain, but an improvement in her mood. We did deep nutritional testing, food allergy testing, and hormonal evaluations, creating a fundamental basis of wellness so that her brain pain could heal. We also discussed the boundaries that she had not been able to set in her personal life with friends or family and the work that she wanted to do in the world. Like all of us, Samantha needed a light to move toward – like a plant seeking the sun – and I knew that Samantha had many great gifts to give. She cleaned up her diet, started to move more, and focused on how she wanted to parent, befriend, and be a guide for others. A big part of this treatment was also helping her deal with the grief of losing many people close to her over the course of the 5 years leading up to her illness. We were able to wean her off all of her pain medication and, over the next few years, she became, again, an inspirational and active participant in her children's lives.

Today, Samantha can watch her children's games and contribute to her community and help her husband while still attending to her own needs. And even now, if she doesn't pay attention to her need for food or sleep or listens to people who mean her harm – she gets a headache. But now she knows what the headache means, and she manages the pain with non-opioid migraine medications and rest, sleep, and meditation.

While Samantha's condition may seem complex, the principles used to heal her are actually quite simple. The treatment of chronic pain in my practice begins with these steps.

1. Use the BodyWise Protocol on a regular basis to 'listen' to what the body is trying to say to you through pain.
2. Identify exacerbating body postures and activities that can be modified (i.e., non-ergonomic position at work or repetitive strain or lack of physical fitness), and alter them as best you can.
3. Consider manual therapies for malalignments or chronic identifiable inflammation that can be improved with manual therapies (chiropractic, massage, physical therapy, craniosacral manipulation, acupuncture, etc.).
4. Establish a mode of exercise that does not exacerbate pain.
5. Reduce inflammation through:
    *   anti-inflammatory diet
    *   anti-inflammatory supplements and medications
    *   addressing allergies, autoimmune disease, and gut health
6. Address issues of anxiety, depression, or lack of purpose.
7. Identify any medical disorders that may be exacerbating pain.

BodyWise Listening

I cannot emphasize enough how important staying bodywise is during your treatment for chronic pain, even self-treatment. Our bodies are created to constantly adapt to our environment. For example, if I accept a job as a carpenter and begin using my upper body for hammering and holding lumber, my arm and back muscles in those locations will sustain 'microtears' with the increased activity. The body will heal those microtears over time by increasing the volume and strength of the muscles, so that I can continue my work. Our bodies get stronger when we push beyond our usual exercise limits. That said, injuries happen when we push too hard. The truth is, if I started tomorrow as a full-time carpenter at my current strength level, I would no doubt injure my neck or shoulder or arm. I'm not strong enough in those muscle groups to sustain that work and would need to start building those muscle groups before my first day of work to ensure that my body was ready.

You can use the BodyWise Protocol to understand the sources of your pain. But, it is just as important to continue to listen to your body as you try new activities or receive treatments, to be sure that you are adapting your body in a way that builds strength, rather than causing further injury. Being bodywise helps you discern what the limit of 'just enough' is at each moment. This is especially important when you're involved in a group activity, such as a yoga class or a group exercise class. No matter what the instructor directs you to do, you need to listen much more carefully to your own body intelligence, doing what feels safe for your body at that moment.

Modifying Posture and Activity

Identifying dysfunctional postures or repetitive activities that cause chronic pain is essential to helping relieve it. We all do repetitive activities to sustain our lives, whether that's sitting at a desk or swinging a hammer, hoisting babies onto our hips, or mopping the floor. Even how we sit, stand, and walk, if done with poor posture, can contribute to chronic pain. This is particularly true for neck and back pain, wrist pain, nerve pain, and headaches. If you are searching for a professional to help you identify issues with your posture or how you lift or walk, there are plenty to choose from. Physiotherapists, chiropractors, osteopaths, and healing traditions such as Rolfing, Pilates, or Feldenkrais can be key in identifying issues with body posture and movement that can be corrected.

Simple ideas such as 'lift with your legs, not with your back' can prevent injury and reduce pain. Because many women in our workforce are sitting at desks during the day, I cannot emphasize how important your position while working or playing on a computer is to your health. I have had innumerable patients on partial and permanent disability simply from repetitive activities using a computer. The picture (opposite) illustrates the proper positioning of the keyboard and your computer screen and the relationship between your hips, knees, and feet.

It is also worth mentioning that any ability to stand (or even walk on a treadmill if you own a treadmill desk) instead of sitting all day can help enormously with maintaining the flexibility and strength of your back and neck. And although we love the flexibility of having laptop computers or tablets, using them on the couch, the bed, or at a café inevitably leads to poor ergonomics – and risk of pain. Recently, I just had my first patient with repetitive strain of the upper body from using his relatively large iPhone 6 as a television while in bed (shoulders slumped, chest collapsed, back bent over, head bent forward, and hands in cramped position). Try to be conscious of how often your very heavy head (10 to 11 pounds) is leaning over your phone, computer, or paperwork instead of sitting on top of your shoulders and letting your spine support its weight. And look for supports that put your laptop, tablet, or phone in more ideal positions for your body. (The Tablift is a great example of this.)

Using Manual Therapies

If your pain is severe or has been long-standing, it is probably worth seeing a medical specialist. For either acute or severe neck and back pain, or any pain related to an injury, I would recommend going to your GP, who can refer you to a physiotherapist. I would recommend exhausting all other options before using long-term medication therapy (though a short 1-week course of NSAIDs, nonsteroidal anti-inflammatory drugs, can be helpful). Significant interventions, such as epidural injections or surgery, should be considered only when other avenues are exhausted, or it is a true medical emergency.

My personal preference for managing chronic neck and back pain or injury is a talented, reliable chiropractor or an osteopath. Not all physicians trained at an osteopathic medical school (with the designation DO after their names) practise osteopathic manipulation techniques, so you will need

Workstation Ergonomics: Ideal Set-up

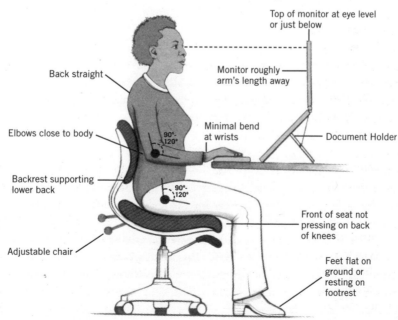

Top of monitor at eye level or just below

Back straight

Monitor roughly arm's length away

Elbows close to body

Minimal bend at wrists

Document Holder

Backrest supporting lower back

Front of seat not pressing on back of knees

Adjustable chair

Feet flat on ground or resting on footrest

90°–120°

90°–120°

to verify this. If nerve pain contributes to the pain that you suffer, you may want to consider acupuncture and traditional Chinese medicine, which can be remarkably effective. Massage is helpful, along with osteopathic techniques such as craniosacral manipulation, for muscular neck and back pain. Keep in mind that the *only* treatment shown to consistently improve long-term back pain is a consistent exercise programme that strengthens core back and abdominal muscles. A physiotherapist or Pilates instructor can help you build strength without hurting yourself. Severe headache syndromes should be diagnosed and treated by a GP. But since headaches can be caused by muscular tension or nerve pain in the neck, a hands-on practitioner (massage therapist, chiropractor, osteopath, craniosacral practitioner) can be helpful in relieving chronic headache pain. And migraines can often be improved with acupuncture.

Chronic pelvic pain needs to be evaluated by a doctor who specializes in women's health, whether gynaecologist, GP, internal medicine, or naturopathic doctor. But once the doctor has addressed any serious medical issues, the most effective practitioners I have found for chronic pelvic pain are the physiotherapists who have advanced training in pelvic floor work. Because these muscles are deep in the pelvis, it is impossible to identify the muscle spasm without a trained practitioner who can feel the muscles. They do this through the abdomen, but also with gentle and careful vaginal touch of the deep pelvic muscles. This may feel uncomfortable, but a skilled and sensitive practitioner can do the work with great sensitivity – and have great results. Other practitioners for chronic pelvic pain include women trained in the Arvigo technique (Mayan abdominal massage), craniosacral practitioners with advanced training in pelvic work, or Chinese medical practitioners with advanced training in *karsai nei tsang* (pelvic energy massage). If you have chronic pelvic pain, finding a practitioner who is credentialled, recommended, and whom you intuitively trust is essential, as the work can be amazingly effective, but is in a very sensitive part of your body.

Finding Exercise for Healing

I do not think it is possible to overemphasize the importance of exercise for anyone with chronic pain. Believe me, I know that many people stop exercising as a result of chronic pain. But movement can heal and restore the body. Every research study on chronic pain, including neck and back pain, all types of arthritis, fibromyalgia, chronic headaches, chronic pelvic pain, chronic abdominal pain, and menstrual pain, shows improvement in pain with some form of exercise.

Exercise can vary from walking to water aerobics to beach volleyball to tai chi or yoga. Yoga practice is remarkably effective at alleviating chronic pain. In fact, yoga is more effective than standard medical care, therapeutic exercise, or even spinal manipulation in relieving chronic low back pain![4] Sometimes, I recommend nothing more than that my patient walk around her house. In Chapter 10, there are exercise options and possibilities for you. But when searching for freedom from pain, it is essential to find natural and creative ways to move your body.

Reducing Inflammation

In holistic medicine, we spend an enormous amount of time helping patients to reduce inflammation in their bodies. Why is this? Inflammation underlies every major illness in the world, including cardiovascular disease, diabetes, musculoskeletal pain, allergies and autoimmune disease, infection, and cancer. Inflammation is caused by the activity of our immune system in fighting off what it believes is an enemy – a virus, bacteria, or parasite. We need inflammation in order to fight off life-threatening infections, but in the modern world, we have many causes of inflammation that are not to our benefit. Poor diet, exposure to toxins, increasing allergy and autoimmune disease, and a chronic stress response all increase the activity of inflammation in our bodies. Pain is the result of the presence of inflammation in muscles, nerves, tendons, and connective tissue. When we take steps to moderate our body's inflammatory response as a whole, we benefit in many ways. We have less pain, but we are also at lower risk for cardiovascular disease, diabetes, and cancer.

The most effective way to reduce inflammation in the body is to change what we put into it. Everything that we eat or drink has a biochemical signal for the body and can turn up or turn down the inflammatory response. Not surprisingly, deep-fried foods, processed foods, hydrogenated oils, sugar, white flour, and red meat all signal the body to increase inflammation. Conversely, fruits and vegetables, especially those that are darkly coloured, as well as legumes and fish signal the body to reduce inflammation. The details of an anti-inflammatory diet are discussed in Chapter 8.

When someone is allergic to a food, medication, or an inhaled or topical chemical product (fragrance, for example), inflammation results. The reaction to these is typically itchy eyes, runny nose, skin rash, or even throat swelling. But I have had many patients who also have increased systemic inflammation, with muscle aching, abdominal pain, or headache. I have seen a patient with daily migraines for 20 years who was literally *cured* by going off gluten; other patients have substantial reduction in their fibro-myalgia pain or arthritis when they identify a food allergy or sensitivity and eliminate the offending food (for more on food allergies and sensitivities, see Chapter 7).

A number of anti-inflammatory compounds that are present in food can be used as supplements to *calm* inflammation. It is advisable to eat (or drink) these natural anti-inflammatory compounds (opposite), although it is also possible to find supplements that contain a combination of these healing plants, to concentrate your intake. These combinations, typically with at least four of the natural anti-inflammatory compounds (opposite), can be found at health food stores or online. Most of them are formulated to relieve chronic pain. These are generally very safe compounds, but, as with any supplements, you should check with your doctor prior to adding them, especially if you are taking a prescription medication.

Turmeric is a potent and important spice from the Ayurvedic, or Indian, healing tradition. It gives the bright orange colour to curry dishes. It con-tains at least two dozen anti-inflammatory compounds – the most widely recognized being curcumin – and has many studies supporting its use in preventing many types of cancer and Alzheimer's disease.[5] It can be eaten with food or consumed in supplement form. I regularly use it to reduce pain in my chronic pain patients.

Green tea is a potent antioxidant with anti-inflammatory properties that has been shown to have a variety of effects, from preventing diabetes, high blood pressure, and cancer to reducing body fat.

Ginger, boswellia (Frankincense), and bromelain are anti-inflamma-tories that are particularly good for arthritis. And fish oil is a powerful anti-inflammatory that reduces pain, among many other benefits, such as reducing triglycerides, improving mood, and making your hair and nails shiny. An anti-inflammatory dose of fish oil is at least 1,000 milligrams of the omega-3's EPA and DHA.

A novel substance used particularly for arthritis is glucosamine. The research on glucosamine is mixed, but enough positive studies are present that I believe it is worth a try, given its safety profile. My clinical experience is that 1,500 milligrams of glucosamine taken daily is quite helpful in about 50 per cent of my patients. It takes 3 to 6 months to determine if glucos-amine will be helpful for you. It's a long time to wait, but if it is effective, it can provide safe, long-term pain relief of a chronic condition. If, in 3 to 6 months, you do not notice any improvement, then it's not the right supple-ment for you.

The other oral treatments for mild to moderate arthritis pain, non-

Natural Anti-Inflammatory Compounds

- Turmeric (curcumin)
- Green tea
- Ginger
- Boswellia (Frankincense)
- Bromelain
- Fish oil

steroidal anti-inflammatory drugs (also known as NSAIDs, including ibuprofen and naproxen), have a wide array of risks, including heart attack, stomach ulcers, and kidney disease. In part, this is because they so specifically and completely block specific aspects of the inflammatory pathway, the COX-1 and COX-2 enzymes. Note that turmeric blocks COX-2 enzymes as well, but much more safely! I do not recommend taking NSAIDs on a regular basis, unless no other good pain relief options exist. I do think that the NSAIDs can be wonderful for acute relief of pain. For example, many women have substantial relief of both tension and migraine headaches with the use of high-dose NSAIDs. I also consider NSAIDs the easiest and most effective treatments for painful periods. Because the menstrual cycle lasts a limited number of days and most women only have pain for a few of those days, it is the ideal circumstance in which to use the powerful NSAIDs rather than opiates such as codeine or hydrocodone, which are less effective, addictive, and mind altering.

A *Time* magazine article on chronic pain in America notes that 100 million Americans have chronic pain and that between 5 to 8 million people use opioids (hydrocodone, codeine, oxycodone, and others) for long-term pain management. The number of prescriptions written for opioid pain medications has skyrocketed in recent years, along with opioid addiction and opioid overdose deaths.[6] We have a crisis in pain management with increasing chronic pain, expensive and often ineffective interventional treatments, and widespread addiction to prescription narcotic medications. Like most medications, prescription narcotics have an appropriate and necessary place in medical treatment. After my tonsillectomy at age 42, I developed a huge affection for my disgusting, tropical-flavoured liquid hydrocodone. The pain of the surgery was so severe that my craving and affection for the substance that relieved the pain grew. As my pain lessened, the disgusting taste of that medication came back to the fore and I stopped using it. But what if I were one of those 100 million Americans in significant chronic pain? Why wouldn't I love and want more of the medication that lessened my pain?

The research shows, very clearly, that exercise, acupuncture, appropriate manipulation, addressing anxiety and depression, healthy diet, and supporting a sense of purpose are all much more effective as a group, with fewer side effects, than chronic narcotics. This is so much the case that the United States Veterans Administration hospitals and clinics are implementing a comprehensive approach to pain that includes all of these procedures for their soldiers, veterans, and families. There are patients in my practice who live with chronic pain on an ongoing basis, for whom narcotic medications are necessary. The pain relief that the medication provides allows them to exercise, visit their loved ones, and do meaningful work in the world. I do not oppose the chronic use of narcotics when all other avenues for treatment have been exhausted, but we want to limit their use as best we can. As with all potentially dangerous treatments, pain medication should be used with caution, and with other procedures, to support someone to have a better life. It is always my great pleasure as a doctor when I get to help the patients be pain-free, off their medications. Because that is helping them to have real freedom, in their bodies and minds.

Addressing Anxiety and Depression

Any treatment of chronic pain would be incomplete without discussing the feedback cycle that extreme stress, depression, and anxiety have with chronic pain. Each one begets the other, with depression and anxiety significantly increasing the risk of pain becoming chronic, and chronic pain itself causing depression. There are good studies showing that psychotherapy is an effective tool for managing chronic pain.

It is not surprising that chronic pain can cause or exacerbate depression, as it often results in a much more limited life. One of the most important offerings I gave to Samantha, my patient suffering from chronic migraines, was the strong belief and hope that her pain could improve. Depression has a way of subtracting hope and instilling an inevitability that the pain will never cease. Part of the healing is to help my patients create a future in which they can do and be what they want, and then reach out for that. (I discuss treatments of depression and anxiety in detail in Chapter 6.) If you experience chronic pain, remember that depression can be a side effect.

Medical Issues That Exacerbate Pain

There are a number of medical conditions that can exacerbate or elucidate the causes of chronic pain. If joint pain is your primary symptom, especially if you are young, the joints are red and swollen, or the joint pain and stiffness occur primarily upon awakening in the morning, it would be important to rule out systemic arthritis. All of us get some form of arthritis, or joint inflammation and damage, if we live past 50. Most of us get wear-and-tear arthritis, called osteoarthritis. It is most common in the knees, hips, fingers, and base of the thumbs. But some women suffer from a systemic arthritis caused by an autoimmune condition. Systemic arthritis can be more serious because it causes substantial joint destruction and it can also be much more painful. It needs to be treated somewhat differently in order to prevent joint destruction, so identification is important. This is relatively easy to do by testing the blood for systemic inflammation with a C-reactive protein (CRP), a rheumatoid factor (RF), and an antinuclear antibody (ANA). If these are positive, then more detailed testing should be done. It is worth noting that infections, such as Lyme disease, can also cause a chronic arthritis syndrome. If you have had tick exposure and have an unusual collection of symptoms that include joint pain, you may want to be tested for Lyme disease and other co-infections.

If your chronic pain is in the form of migraine headaches, you may want to consider hormonal influences, as fluctuating oestrogen levels are common causes of migraine headaches. Testing hormones is not a common practice for most regular doctors, but this is frequently done by holistic physicians or naturopathic physicians. If your migraines are during perimenopause, between 40 and 52 years of age, or if they are always at a particular time in your cycle, such as ovulation or periods, hormone testing that includes oestradiol and progesterone can be helpful. We consider migraines to be one of the many female disorders that is exacerbated by too much oestrogen and too little balancing progesterone. Other disorders in this category are heavy and painful menstrual periods, endometriosis, uterine fibroids, premenstrual symptoms including breast pain, and female cancers such as breast, uterine, or ovarian. By helping to moderate the influence of oestrogen with lifestyle changes, herbs, and hormones, such as progesterone, we can often reduce the frequency and intensity of migraine headaches.

Chronic pain is one of the many conditions that can be improved by having normal vitamin D levels. The majority of women in the United States are actually vitamin D deficient. A normal vitamin D level reduces your risk of autoimmune disease and all types of cancer by 50 per cent, as well as preventing bone loss and osteoporosis. Vitamin D also plays a role in sustaining normal mood. Replacing vitamin D, when deficient, can help to reduce muscle and joint pain. The blood test that you want to ask for is a 25-hydroxy vitamin D. A normal level at most labs is greater than 30 ng/dl. However, if my patient has a high risk of, or currently suffers from, auto-immune disease or cancer, I like to see the vitamin D level closer to 50 ng/dl. I always give vitamin D_3, the active form of vitamin D, as it is universally absorbable. It makes sense to combine it with vitamin K_2 to help ensure that vitamin D is contributing to calcification of a woman's bones, and not the calcification of her arteries or other tissues. If you are not able to have your vitamin D level checked, it is safe to take 1,000 to 2,000 international units (IU) daily. Some women in my practice with exceedingly low vitamin D levels, and a poor ability to absorb vitamin D, can require up to 10,000 international units a day to reach normal levels! Conversely, a healthy, normal woman taking that amount would increase her vitamin D to toxic levels. Because vitamin D is fat soluble and not excreted in the urine, it is very important not to take high levels of vitamin D without having your blood level of vitamin D checked to be sure you have not exceeded the normal range.

As you will hear me say many times in this book, thyroid disease exacerbates pretty much everything. Included among the many symptoms of low thyroid function is muscle pain and joint pain. As we discussed in Chapter 3, be sure that your doctor or holistic therapist checks thyroid stimulating hormone (TSH) as well as your free T4 and free T3, and that your levels are in the optimal range.

Improving Chronic Pain with Your Mind and Heart

Meditation or prayer can be very effective for reducing chronic pain of all types, as well as symptoms of depression or anxiety. As is the case with almost all chronic health conditions, the practice of mindfulness-based stress reduction can substantially reduce pain symptoms, as can transcendental meditation (TM). Just 20 minutes of daily meditation can make a substantial difference in pain. The power of our minds, hearts, and imaginations to shift our physiologies, including inflammation, in beneficial ways, is truly amazing. Much of the research on pain reduction has been conducted on mindfulness meditation, but a number of studies showed similar benefits from other activities, such as prayer, meditative yoga, and walking in nature. Finding these moments of peace creates a pathway where you can make decisions and choose your life independent of the pain, instead of always under the cloud of it.

When I work with patients in my office, I often use a meditative visualization exercise to help them understand and relieve their pain. (See 'Exercise 7: Shifting Pain' overleaf.) When you use your body intelligence to communicate with your pain, and then to begin to soothe it, remarkable things can happen. You may identify an emotional situation or relationship that needs to shift. You may find a visualization that helps you reduce your suffering. Or, you may gain insight into the physiology of the pain itself. You can use the 'Shifting Pain' exercise to help you gain the ability to reduce your pain at will, when necessary.

Given what we know about the power of visualization, I am sure that we are actually reducing the inflammatory mediators at the site of the pain. Remember to check in with your pain more regularly for guidance on how to feel better. Be sure to note if your pain has any messages for you. I work with patients with significant physical pain who, by focusing on the pain sensation and doing visualization exercises, can substantially reduce the experience of their pain.

Use your own body wisdom to guide you to the practices, practitioners, treatments, supplements, exercises, dietary changes, and testing that seem most useful to you, and I am confident that you can find some relief from your chronic pain. Sometimes, our bodies whisper in a language we can barely understand and, at other times, they seem to yell with persistent intensity – as in the case with chronic pain. Listen to trusted sources, and most important, your own body, and let it guide you to a life with less pain and more freedom.

Health Workup for Chronic Pain

A few medical tests that can be helpful in chronic pain:

- C-reactive protein (CRP): to look for chronic inflammation, which may indicate an underlying medical disorder
- Arthritis panel: if significant inflammatory joint pain is the issue – RF (rheumatoid factor) and ANA (antinuclear antigen)
- Thyroid function, as it can exacerbate pain: TSH, free T3, free T4
- 25-hydroxy vitamin D (low levels can cause pain and supplementation can help with pain)

Exercise 7: Shifting Pain

1. Close your eyes if you are able to listen to this exercise on our audio version at doctorrachel.com, in the 'Books' section under BodyWise. For most of us, it is easier to focus inwardly when we are not distracted by what we see outwardly. Otherwise, it is fine to simply relax and read the exercise.
2. Sit or lie in a comfortable position.
3. Take three deep breaths. Breathe in through your nose, allowing your belly to expand, as in the Belly Breathing exercise.
4. Bring your awareness to each part of your body from your toes up to your head, as in the Body Awareness exercise.
5. Focus on an area of your body in which you feel pain.
6. Notice the quality of the pain sensation as in the Quality of Sensation exercise. What type, size, density, temperature, and colour is it?
7. As we did in the Body Feeling exercise, ask your pain, 'What are you trying to tell me?' and listen for or observe a response. After several breaths, move to the next step.
8. Find a relieving visualization for your pain, for example, if the pain is burning and red, imagine that you have a powerful vessel of cooling water that you slowly pour over it. See if you are able to pour enough to begin to cool the pain. If your pain is cold and solid, see if you can warm and liquefy it. If it is dense and hard, see if you can dissolve it or blow wind through it or pull it apart, like a knot of rope. If it is moving like a snake or liquid mercury, find a container to catch it and contain it. Continue to breathe deeply into the area of your pain while you do your relieving visualization. If the pain shifts shapes, shift your relieving strategy.
9. Minimize the size of your pain by imagining that you are gathering it into a box or container, withdrawing it from the far corners of your body with your hands, a tool, or a vacuum cleaner. You can even close the container and lock it. Feel the pain reduce in size and intensity.
10. Now, take a moment to focus on an area of your body that is not in pain. Breathe into the relaxation and flow present in that area.
11. Take a deep breath and give thanks to your body for speaking with you.

CHAPTER 5

Oh Where, Oh Where Has Your Libido Gone?

Libido Quiz

1. Do you feel the desire for sexual activity, either alone or with someone else, at least once a week?

1	2	3	4	5
(Never)	(Rarely)	(Sometimes)	(Usually)	(Almost always)

2. If you are sexually active with yourself or another person, how pleasurable is it?

1	2	3	4	5
(Never pleasurable)	(Rarely pleasurable)	(Often quite pleasurable)	(Frequently very pleasurable)	(Off the charts!)

3. Compared to a time in your life when your sex drive was at its height, how strong is your sex drive now?

1	2	3	4	5
(What sex drive?)	(Significantly less)	(Somewhat less strong)	(About the same)	(The strongest it's been)

4. How often do you feel sexy?

1	2	3	4	5
(Never)	(Rarely)	(Sometimes)	(Usually)	(Almost always)

If you scored:

4–10: low libido

11–15: limited libido

16–20: active libido

**Add the numbers of your answers.
Your Libido score is: _____**

Lack of sex drive may not be the most dangerous medical problem in my office, but it sure causes a lot of distress, and it is *very* common. I have been writing and teaching about healthy sexuality for decades, and consistently, the number-one sexual concern of my students and my patients is a lack of desire. When the body is depleted, there is not enough life energy to accomplish all of our tasks. We use our energy for the things we have to do, and then there is not necessarily enough energy left for the things we want to do – like sex. Or organizing our photos. Or creating a filing system. In this chapter, we'll focus on sex.

I would define low libido as a lack of spontaneous desire for sex (alone or with another), including sexual thoughts and fantasies. My guess is that any doctor who is willing to ask her patients about their sexual desire will find the same result – low libido is the number-one sexual complaint among women. The National Health and Social Life Survey found that, in the United States, one-third of women complain of a lack of interest in sex.[1] The Global Study of Sexual Attitudes and Behaviours (GSSAB) found that 26 to 43 per cent of women experienced low sexual desire worldwide.[2] As both a doctor and a woman, I find this alarming, since satisfying sex has so many benefits – it can be a positive force for health, producing important chemicals in our bodies and important bonds in our relationships. So why are so many of us lacking in desire?

If you were sitting in my office concerned about having low sex drive, you would see me make a large circle with my hands and arms, while saying, 'Libido for women lives in the complex web of our lives and is influenced by our past experiences, our general health, our current relationships, and our hormonal balance.' In other words, women don't separate sex from any other important part of their health and well-being. Which, honestly, is as it should be. Sexual desire is an expression of vibrant health, of creative fire. And we all deserve to have a life that supports that vibrant expression of life-affirming desire.

Here are some of the factors that can cause trouble with your libido:

1. Social and cultural influences
   * Religious
   * Familial
   * Body image
2. Trauma and bad sex
3. Painful sex
4. Hormonal and medical influences

5. Stress and busyness
6. Relationships

One of the more amazing stories of 'libido reclamation' in my office involved a quiet and determined 60-year-old patient of mine, Casey. She had married her husband as a virgin at age 34. She said they had an okay sex life; as we talked, she told me that she never experienced wanting sex, nor did she ever have an orgasm. When she became pregnant with their first child at age 36, her husband said she was fat and unattractive, and he never touched her sexually again. Casey didn't want or miss sex. Her husband apparently had several discreet affairs during their marriage. Casey did not. Now that her child was grown and on her own, her husband wanted a divorce. She agreed.

But amazingly, Casey came to me because she wanted to have a real, satisfying sex life for the first time in her life. She was afraid that she couldn't feel sexual pleasure, because she hadn't been touched for 24 years. I assured her that she actually could have a wonderful sex life, and we started by having her try self-stimulation to orgasm at home and using a mild topical oestrogen preparation to help with vaginal dryness and narrowing. By the end of our work together, Casey had been able to orgasm and, not surprisingly, now looked forward to self-stimulation and penetration. She no longer feels ugly and truly enjoys her body. She has continued her exploration, seeing a sexologist and attending classes and workshops on sexuality, orgasm, and women's empowerment. She is now dating and enjoying fully intimate, sexual life experiences.

It is very difficult to want to have sex if you feel unattractive or unwanted, like Casey. It's also difficult to want sex if sex hurts or is just downright boring, if you and your sex partner are not emotionally connected, or if, like so many women, you're just exhausted and depleted. All of these issues can be addressed and overcome for the large majority of women that I see.

Social and Cultural Influences

The earliest influences on our sexuality are the household and societal sexual norms that we grow up with. If you were raised in a place where most people, for religious or cultural reasons, feel that sex is bad or to be feared, you might suppress your own early sexual exploration. Early fears of sexuality remain with us once we are adults and can be difficult to shake. It is also the case that if you were raised in a family or culture that had strict definitions of what a sexy woman should look like, you may feel inadequate in comparison. Concerns about body image and whether one is desirable enough can kill nascent sexual interest.

I find it infuriating that the image of what is considered sexy in the media is so impossibly out-of-step with what women actually look like. The ability to digitally enhance photographs has only exacerbated this issue. The great majority of potential lovers are interested in you because you are physically attracted to them. Not because you fit some perfect ideal of the female form. Ask any woman-loving man or woman. They like breasts. All breasts. All sizes and shapes. And hips . . . and those lovely derrieres. And particularly in a woman that they care about and find interesting. We can be brutal with ourselves about our bodies, but our lovers typically just want to love us. And in case you were concerned that being overweight might affect your ability to be sexual, real studies of this show that women who are overweight or obese have just as much sexual libido and orgasmic ability as other women.

If it is difficult to overcome all of those voices in your head that keep you from your pleasure (your mum, your priest, your imam, your mean childhood girlfriends, your asshole ex-boyfriend, the magazines in the newsstand), it might be helpful to see a trained sexual therapist. Sexual therapists are experienced in helping you hear the small voice of your desire among the cacophony of other voices blocking the full expression of your passion. They support women in overcoming negative cultural messages, previous traumas, and sexual issues in current relationships. A sex therapist can guide you through a personalized programme of self-exploration and self-discovery so that you can experience your own sexual pleasure. You can find a trained sex therapist through your GP or the College of Sexual and Relationship Therapists (COSRT) or the Institute of Psychosexual Medicine.

Trauma and Bad Sex

The incidence of sexual trauma – incest or rape – before the age of 18 in the United States is similar to the worldwide statistic: 1 in 4 to 1 in 5. In some countries, it is as high as 50 per cent. This is tragic in so many ways. Add to this the number of women having sex too young, sex under the influence, sex that they 'shouldn't' have had, sex that was painful, and insensitive and violating medical pelvic exams – that's a whole lot of women who have had negative sexual and genital experiences. Our genitals are our most private and vulnerable area of our bodies. Of course, trauma can affect any part of our bodies, but when most women experience sexual trauma, they shut down sensations in their genitals and their sexual feelings, in general. Perhaps even while becoming extremely sexually active. This is true for sexual violence, but it can also be true for a woman who has just had bad sex, or has been shamed for being sexual.

Women are smart. We learn from our experiences. And when our bodies have a painful experience, we do a number of things to avoid that pain. We 'shut down' our sensitivity to that area, hoping to numb the pain. We avoid potentially sexual situations entirely, even with ourselves. We turn the pain inward and become depressed or anxious. We gain a lot of weight so that we feel 'sexually invisible.' Or, we try to work out the trauma of our experiences by becoming more sexual, with a variety of partners, sometimes to our own endangerment.

All of these choices are completely understandable, but hard on our sexual selves. The hopeful news is that I have seen the most miraculous, full sexual recoveries in women who have had intense sexual trauma. It is inspiring, and it is possible. If you have had any kind of sexual trauma, I would strongly recommend finding an experienced therapist to help you work out all of the confusing feelings and physical reactions from that trauma. A well-trained psychologist or counsellor can be lifesaving.

Because sexual trauma is not just emotional, it becomes physically present in the body's experience. What I mean by this is that the experience of pain and betrayal can become rooted in the tissues of the area of trauma, in this case, the genitals and other sexual areas of your body. When these areas are touched, it can reenact the physical and emotional experience of the trauma. It is vital to use your bodywise listening while exploring your sexual potential to become aware of when your body is really saying 'yes' and actually saying 'no.'

Sexual trauma happens against our will. The healing process includes developing our abilities to keep ourselves sexually safe. This includes choosing safe partners to be sexual with. It also means choosing not to be sexual when you don't want to. I know that it sometimes seems like indulging your partner's desire and just getting sex 'over with' is not a big deal, but I assure you, it *is* a big deal. When you have sex and don't want to, you teach your body to be touched sexually but to feel numb, and this is the enemy of your desire. We need to respect our body intelligence by only being sexual when our body intelligence says 'yes!' Sexual recovery includes regaining the ability to sense and feel your genital area. To do this, it is vital that you never choose to be sexual when you are numb or don't really want to have sex.

Belly breathing (see page 21) is a helpful exercise when anxiety and fear arise in the process of exploring sexuality. The deep breathing allows the panic reaction to calm and helps you 'reinhabit' your body. For example, if you are beginning to explore self-pleasuring or are experimenting with a partner and you become anxious or afraid, stopping and putting your hand on your belly and taking deep breaths can help you calm your fear. After a few minutes, you can continue, or not, as your body prefers. If you are with a partner, this is a good time to do eye-gazing – sitting or lying facing one another and looking into each other's eyes. It's a simple and lovely way to reconnect and reestablish safety.

The 'Exercise 5: Body Feelings' (see page 34) is essential for listening carefully to what your sexual body is saying to you. For example, if sex is painful, listen to what your body is saying. It could be that you simply need more lubricant, or it may mean that you are feeling too unsafe or scared to have sex. Fully reclaiming your sexual body as your own sovereign territory and releasing the experience of trauma can be miraculously life-giving. This work is sensitive and essential. If you are with a partner, be sure that you communicate clearly when you want to be touched, and how, and the times when you don't. I can't overstate the healing power of open communication. Therapeutic work around trauma is best done with someone trained in the process. I would highly recommend any of the books by Peter A. Levine, PhD, on this topic or a therapist trained in somatic experiencing (see Appendix B).

Painful Sex

I know it seems obvious, but why in the world would someone want to have sex if it hurts? There are a number of reasons that sex can hurt, but a few are so common that they're worth mentioning.

First of all, the most common reason for pain with intercourse or penetration are the hormonal changes of menopause. Menopause is the cessation of ovulation (production of eggs) by the ovaries, resulting in the reduction of oestrogen, progesterone, and testosterone. This occurs naturally with age, typically between 47 and 57. But women can also experience early menopause from surgical removal of the ovaries and/or uterus at any age. Chemotherapy and radiation, typically for cancer treatment, can also severely reduce ovarian production of hormones and induce menopause. Nursing a baby can also induce a menopause-like state of the hormones, because of the suppressive effects of prolactin. So, in addition to the fact that you may have just pushed a baby out through there, the tissues are not so flexible as before, and sex can *hurt*. In natural or artificial menopause, women experience a significant reduction in circulating oestrogen and testosterone, resulting in the vaginal and vulval tissues becoming thinner, drier, and more vulnerable to injury. In this environment, penetrative sex, especially without enough lubrication, can cause many microtears of the vulva and vagina – ouch! I call this vaginal road rash, and it burns and hurts, sometimes severely.

The excellent news is that in almost all cases, this can be ameliorated with topical oestrogens. This is not hormone replacement; it is local oestrogen for the tissues and is safe in all women, with the exception of those who have had breast, uterine, or ovarian cancer. And sometimes, under the careful care of an oncologist, we even use small amounts of vulval oestrogen in cancer survivors. Bioidentical oestrogen, in the form of oestradiol, is readily available by prescription in cream or tablet form for vaginal use. There is also the Estring, a silicone ring impregnated with oestradiol that slowly secretes oestrogen into the vagina in small amounts over 3 months. In addition to oestradiol, there are cream forms of Premarin (conjugated equine oestrogens) for this purpose, but in my opinion, this is an inferior product in that it is created from pregnant horse urine and contains at least 10 conjugated oestrogens, as well as steroids, androgens, and progestogens that are not made in the human body. I prefer that my patients stick to medications or herbs that the body is familiar with and knows how to detoxify.

My favourite form of vulval oestrogen is widely available in Europe. It is oestriol, one of the three oestrogens that our body makes. Oestriol is actually the breakdown product of oestradiol and is helpful for vulval and vaginal lubrication, but is *not* very stimulatory to the breast or uterus, making it, theoretically, a safer product. Even small amounts (1 to 2 milligrams applied to the vulva and/or vagina two to three times a week) can have dramatic effects on the tissue, creating a better lubricated and more resilient vaginal lining. Which makes for happier sex. Oestriol is available on prescription in the UK.

For women who have had breast, uterine, or ovarian cancer there are other options that you can discuss with your physician. Omega-3 fatty acids in the form of flaxseed oil or fish oil taken orally can help with lubrication. Topical moisturizers that are created to stay active, such as Replens or Sylk, are also helpful for many women. Some traditional Chinese medicine-based formulas can also help with vaginal health. And there is some promising research on a hops gel from Germany that helps with vaginal lubrication. In certain cases, it might be safe to consider small amounts of topical hormonal creams, such as DHEA (dehydroepiandrosterone) or oestriol cream or suppository. This, of course, should be discussed with your GP or gynaecologist.

It is worth mentioning that women who go through menopause while remaining sexually active are sometimes just fine without any topical hormones. An active sex life increases the secretion of oestrogen and testosterone, helping with lubrication, and sex itself (with a partner or not) keeps the vulval and vaginal tissues flexible and strong. When women go through menopause without being sexually active, in addition to the changes above, the vaginal opening also shrinks in size, sometimes making pelvic examinations painful. All of these changes are reversible with topical oestrogens and gentle dilation of the vaginal opening with fingers or 'dilators' made for this purpose.

Hormonal and Medical Influences

Perhaps the most important physiological influence on libido is the availability of oestrogen and testosterone. Oestrogen contributes to sexual receptivity – that Marilyn Monroe, hair flip kind of sex drive. But testosterone is the major driver of libido in women, increasing desire for sexual behaviour and increasing genital arousal, sensation, and lubrication.[3] As I have said, sex drive is more than just desire for sex, it is a sign of a passionate life force. And when testosterone is low, in addition to lack of libido and less pleasure, women are tired, less motivated, and have a reduced sense of well-being.[4] In other words, testosterone is a big deal.

To connect all the dots in our exploration of chronic body depletion, guess what reduces testosterone? Adrenal fatigue. Sleep deprivation. Ongoing stress. Depression. And a whole slew of medications. You can see if you are taking one of the sex-offending medications by checking the table of medications in Appendix A, but for most, the path to a better sex life is the path out of chronic body depletion. Almost all of my patients can get the pleasure they want and deserve by working on their fundamentals of health: eating, sleeping, moving, loving, and making meaning (see Chapters 8 through 12).

And sometimes, to be honest, a girl just needs a little help along the way. As testosterone levels diminish with age, it is common for women around menopause to have low testosterone. It is also the case that any woman who has lost ovarian function due to surgical removal of the ovaries or has had radiation or chemotherapy damage has half the testosterone level of a woman who still has her ovaries, even if she is menopausal. Because of this, Europe has approved a 'woman-sized' testosterone patch for the treatment of low libido in these women. In the United States, it is common practice to prescribe testosterone cream formulated at a compounding pharmacy for them. I also use testosterone replacement with my perimenopausal and menopausal patients with low blood levels of testosterone, or levels that are in the low range of normal. If you have a history of breast, uterine, or ovarian cancer, of course, be careful with any type of hormone treatment, including testosterone.

If you are concerned that you have low libido in part due to low testosterone levels, be sure to ask your doctor to measure both free and total testosterone, or total testosterone and SHBG (sex hormone binding globulin), to see if your testosterone is in the low or low-normal range (meaning, it's in the normal range, but below the 50th percentile of normal).

In addition to low levels of oestrogen and testosterone, any chronic illness or chronic pain will reduce sex drive. Specific culprits to look for include (surprise!) adrenal fatigue and hypothyroidism, as well as eating disorders. All of these affect the normal production of sex hormones.

A new medication, Addyi or flibanserin, entered the US pharmacopoeia in 2015 for the treatment of libido in women. It has the serious side effects of low blood pressure, dizziness, and fainting, and is available only under a restricted programme. I cannot recommend the use of this as its effectiveness is small and the risks are significant. There is an interesting combination topical oil on the market, Zestra, that has some broad research showing increased sexual desire and arousal with use. It is applied to the vulval area before sex, with the effects starting in 3 to 5 minutes and peaking in 10 minutes. It is notable that 15 per cent of women experience some burning from it, despite the ingredients being quite safe: borage seed oil, evening primrose oil, angelica root extract, and *Coleus forskohlii* extract. It is available online direct from the manufacturer.

Another potential treatment for low libido that is available in Europe, though not in the United States, is tibolone. Tibolone is a steroid that breaks down in the body into oestrogen. It acts much like hormone-replacement therapy, reducing hot flushes and vaginal dryness. But, interestingly, it reduces SHBG (sex hormone binding globulin), which increases free testosterone levels. This is probably why it also helps with libido. It is an interesting treatment, but comes with all the risks of a synthetic oestrogen (potential increase in breast cancer, uterine cancer, heart attacks, stroke, and blood clots). Still, if you are a menopausal, European woman with low libido, it might be a good fit.

Stress and Busyness

Because we are complex beings, we can have plenty of testosterone, be comfortable with our bodies, have great sexual partners, and *still* have no sex drive. My observation is that many women are, literally, too busy for sex. Which is very sad, as sex, if you pay attention to your body and cultivate your sex drive, gives back in spades what you put into it. Sexual activity (including self-pleasuring) reduces mortality and rates of illness, improves your hormonal profile, and substantially reduces the risk of depression. But your sex drive is like your rejected cat who doesn't want you if you don't want her. You have to give some time and attention to pleasuring your body for your body to spontaneously and lusciously crave pleasure. If you drop into bed after a day of grinding work or parenting where you forgot you even had a body, and expect your sex drive to just be there waiting for you, remember the cat metaphor. Your sex drive turned on her tail and walked off in the opposite direction.

Here are the keys to inviting your sex drive back into your life and your body. Use your body, physically, on a regular basis. Walk, bike, hike, dance the tango, or play badminton. Be active and in your body. Do your body-wise listening so that you can hear what your body is telling you. Eat or rest when needed. Get enough sleep; fatigue may be the number-one killer of sex drive for the average female. Make time for pleasure. This is a big one. If you don't fit sex, with yourself or with another, into your schedule, it will not spontaneously appear. You can see the tail of your rejected sex drive passing around the corner. One of the ways to invite sex back into your life is to use fantasy in ways that are fun. This could be spontaneously imagined fantasies, romance novels, erotica, erotic films, or role play. Letting your fantasy life flourish is a fast way to stoke your libido. Try not to judge what you find sexy. What we fantasize about and how we act in the world are two completely separate things.

It is worth mentioning that some of us are still labouring under the mistaken assumption that it is our partner's job to know what we need sexually and 'give' us orgasms. I can tell you that there is nothing further from the truth. As my mother-in-law once said, 'Everyone is responsible for their own orgasm.' True words. You need to explore yourself so that you know what you like and how you need to be touched to experience pleasure. And then you need to communicate that to your partner, in detail, with your words, your hands, and your sounds. Women and sexuality are *complicated,* and you need to help your partner give you what you want and need. Self-pleasuring is good for everyone and very important for increasing sex drive. And self-pleasuring actually *increases* the frequency of partnered sex. Because libido, like many aspects of the body, has a positive feedback loop. You make time for self-pleasure and increase the number of sexual thoughts that you have, and you are more likely to want to have sex again sooner. Sex begets sex. So put it on your calendar, and make it happen.

Relationships

I have often said, 'Sex is just a mirror of the relationship itself.' And after decades of working with couples, I really believe that to be the case. If you do not want to have sex because you are mad at your partner, it has nothing to do with your health or being rested or having enough testosterone. It has to do with your relationship. And contrary to what you may have seen in novels or movies, fighting and lack of trust do not lead to a better sex life. Trust is the number-one ingredient necessary for a happy, healthy sex life. If you do not trust your partner, either emotionally or physically, it will be very difficult to have a hot sexual life. Exploring the relationship and trying to establish trust is the fundamental piece necessary to support your libido.

If you are struggling with your partner in any significant way, attending to those issues with honesty and compassion is the surest way to reawaken erotic sparks. This is easy to write about but challenging to do! I have been privileged to work with John M. Gottman, PhD, and Julie Schwartz Gottman, PhD, on two relationship books, and their qualifications and success in the field of relationships are unparalleled. You may want to start with one of their books, or explore the opportunities at the Gottman Institute (see Appendix B and gottman.com/couples/private-therapy). Or it might be a boon to your relationship to seek out a couples' therapist. Personal recommendations from friends or a health provider generally work best for finding a therapist you both like, but I have listed resources to find therapists in your area in Appendix B.

Health Workup for Low Libido

- Optimal thyroid function: TSH, free T3, free T4
- Adrenal testing if stress is an issue: salivary cortisol measurements with an integrative doctor
- Total and free testosterone levels, or total testosterone and sex hormone binding globulin (SHBG)
- Consider other hormone testing if you are perimenopausal, menopausal, or have stopped having periods for unknown reasons: oestradiol, progesterone, DHEA-S.
- If you have pain with sex, a good gynaecologic exam should be able to identify any skin conditions or infections contributing to the pain.

I have had the pleasure of seeing women at all stages and ages, with a wide variety of experiences, find their libido and pleasure, even after years of losing it. It is absolutely possible for you to feel that tingly, life-giving rush of sexual pizzazz in your body as well. Be compassionate with yourself, be patient, and don't be afraid to start today.

CHAPTER 6

Wired and Tired:
Relieving Depression and Anxiety

Depression and Anxiety Quiz

1. Do you have little pleasure or interest in doing things?

1	2	3	4	5
(Never)	(Rarely)	(Sometimes)	(Usually)	(Almost always)

2. Do you feel down, depressed, or hopeless?

1	2	3	4	5
(Never)	(Rarely)	(Sometimes)	(Usually)	(Almost always)

3. Do you have trouble concentrating on tasks, such as reading, working on your computer, or watching television?

1	2	3	4	5
(Never)	(Rarely)	(Sometimes)	(Usually)	(Almost always)

4. Do you feel unhappy about where you are in life, personally or professionally, or that you are a failure or have let yourself or your family down?

1	2	3	4	5
(Never)	(Rarely)	(Sometimes)	(Usually)	(Almost always)

5. Do you feel nervous, anxious, or on edge, or do you worry a lot?

1	2	3	4	5
(Never)	(Rarely)	(Sometimes)	(Usually)	(Almost always)

(continued)

Depression and Anxiety Quiz (*cont.*)

6. Do you experience twitching, trembling, shortness of breath, palpitations, tingling, numbness, or shaky feelings?

1	2	3	4	5
(Never)	(Rarely)	(Sometimes)	(Usually)	(Almost always)

7. Are you restless, and do you have trouble relaxing?

1	2	3	4	5
(Never)	(Rarely)	(Sometimes)	(Usually)	(Almost always)

8. Are you afraid of what awaits you in the future?

1	2	3	4	5
(Never)	(Rarely)	(Sometimes)	(Usually)	(Almost always)

Add the numbers of your answers for questions 1–4 (depression).

Your Depression score is: _____

If you scored:

4-8: minimal risk of depression

9-14: moderate risk of depression

15-20: significant risk of depression

Add the numbers of your answers for questions 5–8 (anxiety).

Your Anxiety score is: _____

If you scored:

4-8: minimal risk of anxiety

9-14: moderate risk of anxiety

15-20: significant risk of anxiety

At first glance, anxiety and depression may seem like different, even opposite problems. Anxiety is characterized by feelings of tension, worried thoughts, and physical changes like increased sweating, rapid heartbeat, or elevated blood pressure. Depression, on the other hand, is experienced as sadness, a lack of interest or pleasure in daily activities, feelings of worthlessness, and a lack of energy. Although they can occur separately, most women in my practice experience anxiety and depression hand-in-hand – they're anxious and worried, perhaps unable to sleep or feel calm, and, at the same time, they feel sad and lack energy. In holistic medicine, we call this the wired-and-tired problem.

Tamara is a fit, tanned, well-dressed, affluent 54-year-old with long brown hair and blue eyes, who, from the outside, appears to have it all. Yet, when I first met Tamara, she seemed scared and vulnerable as she sat in the large brown chair in my office. She was new to my practice and was having a recurrence of both anxiety, which was palpable in the room, and depression. Tamara had been an at-home mum for most of her adult life and had a history of significant, years-long depression in the past, where she couldn't get out of bed in the morning. She had been doing fairly well in the past few years, but recently began having a midlife crisis in her marriage, with she and her husband growing apart, fighting, and trying to decide whether they could stay together. At the same time, her now-young-adult son and daughter were struggling with drug use and motivation issues.

Tamara experienced daily anxiety, worry, and insomnia along with hopelessness and uncertainty about her life and her future. Having spent her life serving her family, she was unsure what her next phase should be and the uncertainty in her marriage, parenting, social life, and potential career was overwhelming. In her desperation around her marriage, her kids, and her own deepening depression, she sought help from a therapist and also from me. When we met, she told me that, over the years, she had been on seven different antidepressants with significant side effects and no real improvement and was not interested in trying any of them again. With her new therapist, she was focusing on understanding what she, outside of her family, wanted to do in the world.

Tamara had also lost weight due to lack of appetite, and her beautiful face was gaunt. I asked her to eat every 3 hours with an emphasis on healthy fats (such as avocados, nuts, and olive oil) and protein – both of which help maintain normal blood sugar and thus reduce the anxiety response. When we don't eat for a prolonged period of time, say 4 to 6 hours, our blood sugar drops, and we experience more shakiness, irritability, and anxiety. I think of this as the body's kick in the ass to get up and go find some food! And Tamara needed to listen to her body's call for more nourishment. On my encouragement, she began a regular exercise schedule, which included hiking and yoga. Aerobic exercise is extremely effective for both anxiety and depression – as effective as Zoloft. And meditative exercise, such as yoga or tai chi, is a wonderful treatment for anxiety.

We also started some complementary supplements to support mood: 5-hydroxy tryptophan (5-HTP), St. John's wort, lavender oil, vitamin B-complex, and fish oil. Vitamin B-complex supports adrenal function during anxiety and can also help with depression. Omega-3 fatty acids, such as fish oil, help ameliorate depression and anxiety. Lavender oil has long been used as an aromatherapy calming agent, and, in this case, we were using a unique product which was micronized lavender oil in capsules to take by mouth for anxiety. It is nonaddictive and remarkably effective. St. John's wort is the best-researched antidepressant herb for mild to moderate depression and is used as a first-line treatment in countries like Germany to treat depression. The supplement 5-HTP is the chemical precursor to serotonin – that important neurotransmitter involved in anxiety and depression, which most antidepressants increase in order to treat depression and anxiety. Taking 5-HTP orally increases serotonin production in the body gently, with few side effects, and can help with both anxiety and depression.

Tamara responded remarkably well to these small adjustments, with reduced anxiety, improved sleep, and a greater sense of agency in her life. She and her husband are figuring out how to update their marital agreements in their post-child life stage, and are finding a road map to a new relationship together. She is now training to become a healing practitioner herself, which, not surprisingly, is giving her the sense of purpose she was so desperately missing when she first walked into my clinic. Like many of us, Tamara sometimes struggles to put herself first, and when she stops exercising, or taking her supplements, depression can creep back in. But she now knows how to treat herself – to listen to her body wisdom, and get herself back to yoga and taking what she needs.

Tamara found her way out of anxiety and depression by engaging with what her body and soul needed after a lifetime of ignoring her needs. Her list of interconnected needs included healthy food, sleep, exercise, psychotherapy, honesty in her marriage, and finding a sense of purpose. She was assisted by a number of supplements, but these were not the secrets of her success. The key to her healing was to learn how to listen deeply to her own body and to take the time to give herself what she needed.

Tamara is anything but an isolated case. At some time in their lives, 10 to 20 per cent of women will experience depression, compared to only 8 to 10 per cent of men. Why is this? Most studies examine the impact of hormones and life situations that differentiate men and women, but I think the evidence is fairly clear that women experience anxiety and depression disproportionately because the roles that they are expected to fill require so much giving to others that it sometimes comes *at the expense of their own well-being*. Men who are married to women, whether the marriage is good or bad, live longer than men who are not married, because *women love them and take care of them*. Here's what's even more interesting: Women married to men, as a group, live shorter lives than single women, but women who are in a really *good* marriage live longer than single women *and* are less at risk for depression. Women in a bad heterosexual marriage have *seven times* the risk of depression. It doesn't need to be this way.

The risk factors that predispose women to both anxiety and depression are very similar: being married, especially if it is a bad marriage; having young children or a large number of children (even more so if you are a single parent); struggling financially; having a low-status or high-stress job; lower levels of education; or any history of physical or sexual abuse. Our roles as wives and mothers, and our work in high-stress environments as well as low-status employment, make us less healthy mentally and physically. The roles of wife, mother, and worker all require that women ignore their body intelligence in order to serve others. It is clear from the research that giving to others can also be its own source of mental well-being, but the costs can outweigh the benefits, if you have to take on too much. And, honestly, how many women do you know who are *not* doing too much? Doing more than we can reasonably handle is a plague of modern society.

As I sit in front of my six to-do lists, which are helping me organize all of my current roles – wife, mother, doctor, writer, board member, organization cofounder, and homeowner – I realize that I do not have a list for my *own* body's needs – although I am doing my best to care for myself in the process. Note to self (and new to-do list started)! There is no doubt that all of my roles make it more challenging to focus on my own body wisdom. How to take my own needs and desires seriously among all the demands of the people and the work that I love is an ongoing conversation. I find myself asking myself while I write: Am I hungry? How is my neck while typing? Do I need a nap? I am literally writing a book on body wisdom, and I still have to remind myself to do these self-checks at regular intervals; otherwise I would lose sight of my own needs.

Depression, Anxiety, and Health

Depression and anxiety take an enormous toll on us. Depression increases the risk of a heart attack to almost three times the normal risk – twice the increased risk attributed to smoking, hypertension, or diabetes; it literally hurts our hearts. A diagnosis of depression makes the elderly (over 65) have a 60 per cent increased risk of mortality.

So what are we doing to help women who are anxious or depressed? Well, one in four women in the United States now takes a psychiatric medication.[1] *One in four.* I am not opposed to wisely using psychiatric medications: I am someone that sometimes gladly prescribes antidepressants to a woman with severe, debilitating depression, anxiety, or suicidal thoughts. But we have to consider the impact of all of those prescriptions. Almost all antidepressants flatten mood – that is, they improve your lows, but they also reduce your highs – making life just a bit more bland, without its normal ups and downs. They also commonly reduce libido and orgasmic ability, which is depressing in and of itself – particularly given that sex can improve both anxiety and depression.

But how effective are antidepressants? A meta-analysis of all antidepressant studies from 1990 to 2009 showed that there was significant improvement in depression *only* in the most severely depressed group, which constitutes only about 13 per cent of all depressed patients. The effect of antidepressants on mild to moderate depression was *nonsignificant*.[2, 3] Meaning, the participants were as likely to improve by chance as they were from taking antidepressants. And in the largest study of major depression ever done, antidepressant effectiveness with the first medication tried was initially 37 per cent, with a relapse rate within the first year of 40 per cent.[4] Patients who didn't respond were escalated to additional and alternate medications. The drop-out rate, despite the provision of free, high-quality care, was 42 per cent, which says something about the side effects *and* the lack of effectiveness. After all interventions, the number of patients who were still in the study, and in remission from depression at the end of 1 year, was *15 per cent*. Not an impressive number. And if you take into account the number of patients who dropped out of the study, the percentage of the 4,041 patients who were relieved of depression through medication treatment by the end of the study was 2.7 per cent. Honestly, a new puppy could have done a better job.[5]

Innovative Approaches to Depression and Anxiety

1. Confiding in and getting support from someone you trust
2. Meditation or any contemplative spiritual practice or biofeedback
3. Exercise in any form
4. Healthy, anti-inflammatory diet
5. Omega-3 fatty acids
6. Restful and refreshing sleep
7. Light therapy, vitamin D, and 5-HTP for seasonal depressive symptoms
8. B vitamins for mood support
9. Mitochondrial support for depression: SAM-e and creatine
10. Herbs for depression and anxiety: St. John's wort, lavender, L-theanine, valerian, and kava
11. Acupuncture and hormones: DHEA, thyroid, oestrogen, and progesterone

So what are we to do? I still prescribe antidepressants when patients are desperate and in distress: severe depression with suicidal thoughts, severe panic disorder, and debilitating anxiety. And I do my best to optimize all of the other approaches to depression and anxiety in these patients, so that we can limit the number of medications, the strength of the medications, and the amount of time that they have to be on them. With patients who have mild to moderate depression or anxiety, I use a variety of other, generally safer, tools. I have even prescribed a new puppy a time or two.

Not surprisingly, just as depression can cause medical illness, such as a heart attack, medical illnesses can cause or contribute to depression. It is important to test for thyroid disease, as it is so common and can cause depressive symptoms. Also, significant anaemia can also make us feel sluggish, tired, and depressed, and it's easy to test for. And, if you are particularly exhausted, adrenal testing might also be in order. It can be useful to test for normal B_{12} and vitamin D levels as well. The details for all of the suggested laboratory tests for depression and anxiety are in the box at the end of the chapter for you to share with your health practitioner.

As depressing as the data on antidepressants is, there is hope! Many studies show the decent efficacy of simple, safe behavioural treatments for depression. And data continues to accumulate that supports the use of various herbs and supplements. Here are some of the innovative ways that we are successfully approaching anxiety and depression.

Confiding In and Getting Support from Someone You Trust

The first questions that I ask my patients who are suffering from anxiety or depression have to do with understanding their social support and the strength of their relationships with their loved ones. Loneliness, not surprisingly, increases depressive symptoms significantly; it increases two of the other symptoms of body depletion as well: pain and fatigue.[6] If you are suffering from depression or anxiety, one of the first recommendations I give is to spend more time with someone who can help you understand your pain, whether a loved one or a good therapist. Being able to confide in a spouse, a sibling, a parent, a good friend, or a professional can literally be lifesaving. Finding time to talk honestly with someone you trust about your feelings is enormously important. We are human animals, and we are created to live in a tribe. Human touch and interaction, when safe and kind, improve our health and well-being at every level.

If you need further support, finding a skilled therapist to whom you can relate can be lifesaving. Some women think that going to therapy means that they are weak, or that they carry a stigma of being mentally ill. Nothing could be further from the truth. I am the woman that I am, and capable of doing what I do, in part because of the personal work that I've done in therapy. It's a huge gift to yourself to take your emotional needs seriously enough to get the help you need. When you're looking for a therapist, or any practitioner, for that matter, remember that your comfort and trust in that practitioner are paramount. This is a key moment to use your body intelligence to help you feel the rightness of the fit with this person. Your connection to your therapist, doctor, or practitioner has an enormous impact on how successful the treatment is for you. You wouldn't marry just any nice, qualified guy or gal – it has to be the right person for *you*. Similarly, you may meet with a perfectly capable therapist who just isn't a good match for you. It's not a criticism of her work to leave the therapeutic relationship, just a lack of fit. Be sure that you find a clinician you can relate to, that you feel safe with. The kind of deep work that is possible when you work with someone you inherently trust is beautiful and breathtaking.

Meditation, Contemplative Spiritual Practice, or Biofeedback

In 2015, a systematic meta-analysis examined all randomized, controlled trials (in other words: really well-done studies) that were available on spiritual practice and health. The results showed substantial improvements in both depression and anxiety using a variety of spiritual and meditative practices. When a patient comes to see me with symptoms of depression and anxiety, I always ask if she already has a religious or spiritual practice. Using sources that feel sacred and meaningful *for you* is the key here. Which may mean that you embrace your childhood religion, or not. You may pick another tradition that you love, such as yoga with meditation, or pagan ritual, or Sufism – or create your own celebratory form of spirituality. Use your body wisdom to find a practice or tradition that feels right *to you,* that makes you feel calm or joyful inside. You can be a dedicated atheist and still benefit from mindfulness meditation, which is intentionally secular.

From a health point of view, the particularities of the meditation or spirituality do not matter, as long as the values of compassion, humility, integrity, and reverence for life are present – as they are in all major religions. The keys to the benefits of meditation and spirituality include finding a quiet time to focus inward, breathing deeply (as in our belly breathing practice on page 21), and focusing on something of benefit to you. The Zen Buddhists try to clear the mind and dwell in emptiness. The Tibetan Buddhists focus on finding compassion for self and others. Taoists focus on breathing into and expanding the heart and other invigorating organs. Christians pray for themselves, their families, their communities, and the world at large and ask for help from Jesus or God. Hindus recite mantras, small phrases that focus the mind, such as 'om.' Jews might recite a daily prayer on the oneness of God. Muslims can recite the five daily prayers to Allah.

In mindfulness meditation, we focus on the breath and allow our thoughts to come and go, trying not to react to them. To observe the present moment without judgement. I am currently trying to meditate/pray for 15 minutes three times a week. I would consider this the minimum to feel an effect from the practice. Many teachers believe that daily prayer or meditation, even if short (5 to 10 minutes) is better than longer sessions less often. And like most things, the more you do it, the more benefit you get. Whatever your practice, the point is to relax the mind and body and open your heart. Doing this reduces stress and cortisol levels and helps to ameliorate depression and anxiety.

If you are new to meditation as a practice, there are innumerable sources to learn more about meditation, from books to smartphone apps to courses that may be available right in your neighbourhood. And most religious groups have prayer circles or classes that you can join. Can't just sit and meditate or pray? There are quite a few people in my practice for whom sitting meditation is a special kind of torture. They tend to be creative people with very active minds and bodies, who literally have trouble sitting still. I call them moving meditators. Their minds are quieter when their bodies are engaged, and they tend to do better with practices such as yoga, qigong, or tai chi – moving meditations. A simple form of this would be walking meditation, walking in nature while breathing intentionally or repeating an inspirational phrase with each step.

Another option for those who have a hard time engaging their own thoughts and minds is guided meditation. I first experienced a version in medical school 25 years ago, written by the grandfather of guided meditation, Martin Rossman, MD. I used that meditation for years, to bring me peace in the chaos of my medical training. The beauty of guided meditation is that another voice leads you through a series of visualizations – which are proven to reduce anxiety and depression. Dr Rossman has a variety of guided meditations to choose from, including some for anxiety and depression, on his website (thehealingmind.org). And if you just want to try some, there are a number of good guided meditation smartphone apps available.

If you are a visual person or are more engaged by scientific feedback, you may appreciate the biofeedback system of HeartMath. Biofeedback works by monitoring your body and giving you visual or auditory feedback on bodily metrics, such as your heart rate or body temperature. The HeartMath method now has decades of research supporting its use in multiple settings to reduce stress and cortisol levels, calm anxiety, and reduce depressive symptoms.[7, 8] In one study, there were improvements in mental and emotional well-being in more than 5,500 people in just 6 to 9 weeks, including a 50 per cent drop in fatigue, a 46 per cent drop in anxiety, and a 60 per cent drop in depressive symptoms. A HeartMath user places a small clip on her ear or finger that monitors her heart rate. The HeartMath algorithm captures not just the heart rate itself, but the variability in the heart rate over time. In a state of calm or happiness, the heart rate varies in a predictable sine-wave curve, a gentle undulating wave. In a state of anxiety or anger, the heart rate varies in a jagged way that resembles treacherous mountain peaks. By using deep breathing, tuning into one's heart, and creating a memory of a love-filled time (is this sequence beginning to sound familiar yet . . . ?), the user learns to recreate the sine-wave, coherent heart rate pattern. HeartMath has visual programmes that work on a smartphone, a computer, or even a small independent iPod-like device that you can carry with you. Using HeartMath biofeedback in the morning and at lunch or at the end of the day helps us maintain that ideal, calm-but-alert state of being that the coherent heart rate pattern reflects. To learn more about HeartMath, go to Heartmath.com. Some NHS services use this in their psychology departments.

Exercise, Healthy Diet, Omega-3s, and Sleep

There is literally *not one* depressed or anxious patient who gets out of my office without a serious consideration of how and when she is going to exercise. This is because exercise is *so* effective for mild anxiety and depression – just as effective as any antidepressant, and with much better side effects. In a study of patients with major depression that compared exercise with sertraline (Lustral), patients improved with both treatments at 4 months, but at 10 months, far more of the sertraline patients had recurrent depression, whereas the exercising patients remained in remission. They continued to be free of depression.[9] In other words, exercise works *better* long-term than SSRI antidepressants (like sertraline), even for major depression. The ideal exercise for depression and anxiety involves an aerobic component, meaning that you are breathing hard when you do it. Think running, walking briskly, cycling, swimming, dancing, using a treadmill or stair-climber, or playing most sports. Ideally, you want to exercise at least 5 days a week for 30 minutes each day, but anything helps! Details on finding the best exercise for you are in Chapter 10. Exercise could be the most important intervention you have for your general mood. It is that effective.

It isn't surprising that diet affects your mood. Most of us use food for comfort from sorrow, for celebration, for expressions of love, or for simple joy. It is human to have emotions about food. What is interesting here is that certain foods can *cause* fatigue, sadness, or anxiety. While many people have individual reactions to certain foods – unreasonably hyped on caffeine or high on sugar – there are certain generalizations about food that have relevance to your mood. A study in Tehran showed that the more processed food young adults consumed, the more likely they were to be anxious.[10] Eating an anti-inflammatory diet rich in dark-coloured fruits and vegetables, whole grains, legumes, and healthy fats, such as olive oil or avocados, reduces your risk of depression. Inflammatory foods to limit include processed foods, especially those with hydrogenated oils, which are highly inflammatory, fried foods, and sugar. Using anti-inflammatory compounds, such as turmeric (or curcumin) or omega-3 fatty acids (commonly taken from fish oil) may also improve depression in some patients.

I routinely put my depressed and anxious patients on 1,000 milligrams of the omega-3 EPA, preferably in combination with at least 500 milligrams of DHA. Of course, eating fatty fish several times a week is also a great approach, as long as you are careful about choosing fish that is low in mercury and toxins. In fact, fish consumption correlates with lower risk of depression.[11]

And you will probably not be surprised to learn that good sleep is critical in this, as well. Research clearly shows that a lack of sleep increases

Seasonal Affective Disorder is characterized by:

- Depression that starts in autumn or winter
- Carbohydrate cravings
- Afternoon slumps with decreased energy and concentration
- Decreased interest in work or other activities
- Increased appetite with weight gain
- Increased sleep and excessive daytime sleepiness
- Lack of energy
- Slow, sluggish, lethargic movement
- Social withdrawal

depression and anxiety, not to mention every single symptom of chronic body depletion, which is why we give sleep its own chapter a little later.

Light Therapy, Vitamin D, and 5-HTP for Seasonal Symptoms

Some of us seem to struggle with depressive symptoms more during the winter months. Much of this is from the decreased light exposure because of shorter days and more time spent indoors. When the depressive symptoms are significant, it is called seasonal affective disorder, or SAD, which is described in the box on the previous page.

Does not sound like much fun, does it? As if we needed any more carbohydrate cravings during the Christmas holiday season!

Luckily, there are very specific strategies to help with SAD. The best prevention and treatment is increased exposure to light – preferably natural light. So when the weather is nice (or even if it isn't) try to spend some time outside absorbing the sun's rays. Sunlight directly stimulates your brain through the retina at the back of your eyes, impacting the production of melatonin and neurotransmitters that affect sleep and mood. It can also be very helpful to be exposed to full-spectrum indoor light during the day. You can obtain full-spectrum lightbulbs, either incandescent or fluorescent, in all sizes and shapes at lighting stores or online. And for significant symptoms, a full spectrum lightbox can be very effective (see below).

Finding a Lightbox for SAD

For those with seasonal affective disorder (SAD), ordering a professionally designed lightbox that produces at least 2,500 lux but can go up to 10,000 lux at eye level can be very effective. Exposure to 2,500 lux for 2 hours daily or to 10,000 lux for 30 minutes daily seems to be equally effective. The lightbox should be placed on a desk or table so that the light easily enters the eyes, without the need to gaze directly at the light source. It usually takes a week or two to know if the therapy will be effective in lifting depressive symptoms. And recently, research studies have shown that even depressed people without seasonal affective symptoms benefit from light therapy. In a three-armed study, fluoxetine had a nonsignificant effect on depression, light therapy alone showed significant improvements in depression, and the two together showed the largest improvements in depression.[12]

Maintaining adequate vitamin-D levels may also be helpful in preventing or treating SAD. Studies have found a decrease in central serotonergic activity in patients with SAD. We can naturally increase serotonin levels in the body by supplying the body with the precursors to serotonin: tryptophan or 5-hydroxy tryptophan (5-HTP). This should always be done in discussion with your doctor, as there can be risks, and these precursors can interact with antidepressants and have potential side effects.

I typically start with 100 milligrams of 5-HTP before bed and increase by 100 milligrams weekly up to 200 to 400 milligrams, before bed or divided twice daily. 5-HTP can also be used for mild depressive symptoms, whether or not one has seasonal affective disorder.[13] There are very few side effects of 5-HTP for most people, but the common one would be that you find it stimulating rather than relaxing. If this is the case, it's either not the right fit, or you should only take it in the morning. Also, since 5-HTP increases serotonin synthesis, it should only be used with serotonin medications (the SSRI and SNRI antidepressants and buspirone) under the care of a doctor. And, like the medications that increase serotonin, 5-HTP can cause some stomach upset.

B Vitamins for Mood Support

We discussed the vital role that the B vitamins play in maintaining energy and preventing fatigue in Chapter 3. Suffice to say that sufficient B vitamins are also absolutely necessary for the maintenance of normal mood. In particular, folic acid is essential, and is even being used by psychiatrists in a specialized form to augment antidepressant therapy (methyl folic acid or methyltetrahydrofolic acid – MTHF). An unusual number of common medications (see box overleaf), including almost all of the antidepressants, deplete folic acid in the body, making it extremely important for you to supplement your diet with folic acid during treatment with any of these medications.

However, the type of folic acid supplementation used in depression matters, because some of us have genetic abnormalities that make us particularly vulnerable to low folic acid levels. I begin to suspect that genetic abnormalities may be present in my patients when there is a lifelong history of depressive symptoms and/or a strong family history of depression.

Because of these genetic errors that slow folate metabolism, some people are slow to make necessary neurotransmitters and are vulnerable to depression and anxiety. We have just begun to test for some of these genes, and the best studied are the MTHFR genes, which are relevant to

Medications That Reduce Folic Acid

- Lamotrigine
- Carbamazepine
- Phenobarbital
- Valproate
- Methotrexate
- Sulfasalazine
- Oral contraceptives
- Metformin
- Niacin
- Fenofibrates
- SSRIs (fluoxetine, escitalopram, etc.)
- Acid blockers (omeprazole, ranitidine, etc.)
- Warfarin

cardiovascular risk, cancer risk, and depression risk. Genetic testing is becoming more common in the US, but it is not common practice here. If there are abnormalities, the risk for depression goes up. And the possibility of being able to reverse some of those symptoms with methyl folic acid increases.[14, 15]

If you have known abnormalities in your MTHFR genes, or if you simply have a strong family history of depression, it may be worth trying a methyl folic acid supplement. I generally start at a dose of 1 milligram, though doses as high as 15 milligrams are used by psychiatrists and are available by prescription. However, it is advisable to always increase the dose slowly. I have seen depressed bipolar patients with significant deficits in their methylation pathways actually become manic on too much methyl folic acid, too fast. The safest way to try methyl folic acid is to start slow (and even slower if you are sensitive!) and increase gradually, staying on the same dose for at least 3 to 4 days before increasing. Methyl folic acid comes in a number of forms, from prescription to over-the-counter supplements. I would also recommend that if you want to try a supplement to increase methylation ability, you also take other important vitamins that aid in methylation, such as methyl B_{12}, B_6, magnesium, tri-methyl glycine, and/or SAM-e (which we'll discuss next). I also always advise taking a B-complex supplement with any single high dose of a B vitamin, to be sure that there is a balanced amount of Bs available for the body.

A novel treatment for depression and anxiety is the sugar alcohol inositol, which is also part of the B vitamin group. It is needed in the body for serotonin synthesis and has been shown to be effective in randomized controlled trials for depression, panic disorder, obsessive compulsive disorder, and bulimia. In fact, inositol at 15 grams was compared to the SSRI fluvoxamine for the treatment of panic disorder and was more effective at 4 weeks, and equally effective at 9 weeks, with fewer side effects. Inositol is a sweet-tasting powder taken at 2 to 6 grams, two to three times daily, and has very few side effects.[16]

All of these are options that you should discuss with your doctor but have been shown to have positive effects on depression.

Mitochondrial Support for Depression

Supporting our intracellular energy factories – our mitochondria – is essential to restoring a normal energy level. Not surprisingly, it turns out to be key to reducing depression as well. S-adenosyl methionine (SAM-e) is an intracellular energy molecule that has been well-studied for the treatment of depression and, interestingly, osteoarthritis. It works well for both. It also has a much faster onset of action than most antidepressants, with full effect within 2 weeks. Because of this, I will often start my depressed patients on a supplement form of SAM-e, while waiting for longer-acting, synergistic antidepressants (like St. John's wort or an SSRI) to fully work. I strongly recommend using SAM-e and all mood interventions, supplement or otherwise, under the care of a knowledgeable doctor. SAM-e is stimulating and can increase anxiety if you are anxious, so start low and go slow. It can also induce mania if you are bipolar, and can interact with antidepressants and some painkillers.

Another mitochondrial energy support is creatine monohydrate, a supplement successfully used by bodybuilders to increase muscle mass. Creatine plays a key role in energy production and fluctuates in the body with the level of depression. A recent trial of women with major depressive disorder shows that creatine monohydrate, taken at 5 grams a day, significantly improves the efficacy of escitalopram (an SSRI) and speeds the response to therapy.[17] You may want to try creatine, along with the other suggestions above, if depression is an issue for you.

Herbs for Depression and Anxiety

Probably the best known herb used to treat both anxiety and mild depression is St. John's wort. It is used first-line in Germany for mild to moderate depression and is well-established as an effective antidepressant – equivalent in effectiveness to prescription antidepressants – with fewer side effects.[18] Like the SSRIs, St. John's wort also has an anti-anxiety effect that is nice for my patients with both depression and anxiety. St. John's wort is my go-to herb for significant depression, and I often combine it with SAM-e for a faster onset of action. The dose of St. John's wort is 450 milligrams twice daily. I typically have someone start on 450 milligrams in the morning for 3 days and then add the afternoon dose if it is well-tolerated. St. John's wort takes 4 weeks to achieve full effect, and its major risk involves interactions with other drugs and supplements. This can make it tricky to use in patients who are taking other medications, and, if you are taking medications, it should absolutely be monitored by your doctor to be sure that there are no toxic side effects. I want to emphasize that St. John's wort decreases the potency of birth control pills – making pregnancy possible, even if you are taking them. It can also decrease the potency of hormone-replacement therapy.

Lavender oil has been used as an inhalant – in sachets, sprays, oils, and lotions – for centuries. The smell induces calm and sleep. Lavender oil is now available in an oral form, collected into microscopic bubbles and placed in a capsule that allows it to cross the intestinal barrier. Once it does, it induces calm and reduces anxiety. It is marketed as Lavela. It's not addictive or dangerous. And the common side effect is belching lavender, which is, well, flowery. But for most people, not terrible. It is my newest favourite anxiety treatment that doesn't make you tired. It can be used as needed – when anxiety arises, or regularly, depending on your needs. It is a frequent visitor in my office for my patients who sometimes struggle with an overly anxious, busy, obsessive mind.

My other favourite treatment for mild anxiety is L-theanine, which is an extract from green tea. It increases GABA and dopamine and causes a calm alertness, without making you tired.[19] I always think of those Zen monks in Japan sipping their green tea with calm alertness. L-theanine also enhances attention, focus, memory, and learning, which is pretty darn cool. This is another frequently prescribed supplement in my office because of its lovely effects and lack of side effects. It can be used at 100 to 400 milligrams up to twice daily on a regular basis, or simply as needed.

Valerian root is my favourite herb for sleep, and the most effective, according to research. It is also a great anti-anxiety herb, but, unlike lavender or L-theanine, it will usually make you tired! It's a good option for more severe anxiety spells and for evening use, when you will no longer be driving or working. Valerian can be taken during the day in very small doses, 20 milligrams or less. In fact, it is widely available in 'sleep teas' at a dose of about 20 milligrams. For sleep, or more severe anxiety in the evening, I use doses as high as 600 milligrams. It is important not to combine valerian with alcohol or other depressant medications.

Acupuncture and Hormones

Acupuncture, which is extremely safe, has been shown to be as effective a treatment for depression as antidepressants, in a meta-analysis (keeping in mind that this is not saying much!).[20] But I would argue that even though the studies are not perfect, acupuncture and Chinese herbs are a safer approach to depression, with far fewer side effects than antidepressants. Acupuncture is also likely to be helpful for anxiety as well.[21] Since acupuncture treats the whole person, it is an ideal procedure for women with chronic body depletion. If you are investigating treatment with acupuncture and herbs, look for a traditional Chinese medicine practitioner (TCM) who specializes in treating women and emotional issues.

As we discussed in Chapter 3, treating adrenal fatigue with DHEA may be helpful for energy, and also for mood. Similarly, in a woman who is perimenopausal or menopausal, using bioidentical hormones can be an amazing balancing treatment for depression and anxiety. Ideally, hormones smooth out the rocky emotional effects of the menopausal transition, helping with sleep, anxiety, and depression. Certainly, not every woman needs hormones, but when your emotional symptoms are poorly affected by hormonal instability and disturbed sleep from hot flushes, hormone replacement can treat the source of the problem. When a woman stabilizes into menopause, we gently wean the hormones down, and, ideally, off. Long-term use of hormone-replacement therapy increases the risk of breast cancer and cardiovascular disease. But using bioidentical hormones, especially when the oestrogen is given through the skin in a patch or cream, appears to be safer than tablets, especially when limited to around 5 years around the menopausal transition for most women. Keep in mind that some women can get through the emotional and physical swings of menopause using herbal support, such as black cohosh or Vitex and others. If your emotional symptoms coincide with perimenopause, menopause, or your premenstrual phase, please see a practitioner (or consult your GP) who can help you find more balance with your hormonal transitions. *The Hormone Cure* by Sara Gottfried, MD, is also a great resource for gaining a deeper understanding of your own hormonal profile and what you can do to optimize your experience. You will find a more detailed discussion of the pros and cons of hormone-replacement therapy in Appendix A.

We've discussed thyroid function throughout this book, because it is key to all of the symptoms of body depletion syndrome. Low thyroid function causes depressive symptoms and high thyroid function can increase anxiety. It is essential to have your thyroid checked if depression and anxiety are issues for you. Also, in a patient whom I am treating for both low thyroid function (hypothyroidism) and depression, I will 'optimize' thyroid replacement, as taking more thyroid medication can have an antidepressant effect. I like to keep the TSH within the normal range, but push the dose of the thyroid medication as high as we can, while keeping the TSH normal. Thyroid replacement, as we've discussed before, includes both levothyroxine (T4) and liothyronine (T3). Most physicians use only T4 to treat low thyroid function, as it converts to T3 in the body. However, some people do not convert T4 to T3 well, and adding T3 to their thyroid replacement can boost mood and energy. You can discuss possibly adding T3 (liothyronine) to your regime with your doctor.

Medications for Depression and Anxiety

I am a doctor who likes what works. And in certain situations, what works is medication. As always, the decision to use medication is a good time to use your bodywise intuition to guide you to what might work for you. I have patients with severe depression who do not respond to any medications. And for them, we use all the other strategies. And I have patients who don't respond to the other strategies, but very quickly respond to medication when they have a depressive episode.

The most commonly prescribed medications for depression and anxiety (including panic disorder and obsessive compulsive disorder) are the SSRIs: selective serotonin reuptake inhibitors. They include fluoxetine, citalopram, escitalopram, paroxetine, sertraline, and fluvoxamine. These are the first-line medications chosen by most doctors. As we've discussed, they can be effective, especially in major depression, generalized anxiety, and panic disorder. Choosing which one is up to you and your doctor, with people having better reactions to some rather than others. Fluoxetine is the most stimulating and works well in someone who suffers from can't-get-out-of-bed depression. Paroxetine is the most sedating or calming, and might be a good choice for someone who is anxious, as is sertraline. The other SSRIs fall somewhere in the middle. Consider adding creatine and a B-complex vitamin, as we discussed above, to increase the effectiveness of your SSRI. It generally takes at least a month to know if your medication is working for you, and most side effects occur in the first several weeks. If the side effects are not too dramatic, it is often worth sticking it out to see if the side effects improve along with your depression or anxiety. Remember that all of the SSRIs have the possible side effects of attenuated mood, fewer highs and fewer lows, and reduced sex drive and orgasmic ability. SSRIs should never be stopped suddenly; it is vital to wean off them slowly and under the care of a doctor.

Bupropion is a unique antidepressant that acts on the dopamine, rather than the serotonin, system. It is an activating antidepressant and thus not appropriate for an anxious patient, but good for someone who has trouble with motivation. It has very few side effects. In fact, it seems to actually improve sex drive in some women. It is used to help with giving up smoking as well. It is a good choice for someone who doesn't respond to other means or who needs additional help with major depression as it can be added to an SSRI or SNRI (serotonin norepinephrine reuptake inhibitor). I tend to choose Bupropion first in a depressed patient who is tired and unmotivated, and not experiencing anxiety.

SNRIs are another class of medication used for both depression and anxiety (including panic disorder and obsessive compulsive disorder). They include venlafaxine and duloxetine. These medications are typically used for

Sample Treatment Protocol for Mild Anxiety

1. Confiding in and getting support from someone you trust
2. Belly breathing for anxiety symptoms
3. Meditation or any contemplative spiritual practice
4. Restful and refreshing sleep
5. Exercise, in any form, at least 30 minutes 4 days a week
6. Healthy, anti-inflammatory diet
7. Fish oil with omega-3: EPA, at least 1,000 milligrams and DHA, at least 500 milligrams
8. L-theanine: 100 to 200 milligrams up to three times daily
9. Lavela (oral lavender oil): 1 capsule daily, as needed
10. For panic disorder or obsessive compulsive disorder, consider inositol 2 to 6 grams, twice daily.
11. Consider valerian root, up to 600 milligrams, 45 minutes before bed, for sleep.
12. Consider adding 5-HTP, 200 milligrams before bed, in consultation with your doctor.

Sample Treatment Protocol for Mild Depression

1. Confiding in and getting support from someone you trust
2. Meditation or any contemplative spiritual practice
3. Restful and refreshing sleep
4. Exercise, in any form, at least 30 minutes 4 days a week
5. Healthy, anti-inflammatory diet
6. Fish oil with omega-3: EPA, at least 1,000 milligrams and DHA, at least 500 milligrams
7. Vitamin D$_3$: 2,000 IU (more if you are very low in vitamin D)
8. Methylated folic acid: 1 to 2 milligrams with a B-complex (and as high as 15 milligrams)
9. Vitamin C: 500 milligrams twice daily
10. Consider SAM-e, 200 to 600 milligrams in the morning or 5-HTP 200 milligrams before bed.
11. In discussion with your prescribing physician, consider St. John's wort at 450 milligrams twice daily or other options.

recalcitrant depression and anxiety that haven't responded to other medications or interventions. They can also be used to help with chronic pain. They have a number of common side effects, including nausea, dizziness, and sweating, which is why they need to be started slowly. Like the SSRIs, they also attenuate mood (reduce the highs) and cause low libido and orgasmic dysfunction. Weaning off an SNRI can be a long and unpleasant process. I recommend very small, incremental reductions in the medication, stabilizing the dose for 2 weeks before reducing it again. Because of the many side effects and the difficulty of the weaning process, I am reluctant to prescribe these unless there is no other alternative.

Mood stabilizers are typically used in patients with bipolar disease, and there are many, from lithium to antipsychotics to antiseizure medications. They can be vital in someone with unstable bipolar disease, but all of them have pretty hefty side effects, some of them dangerous. One of the newer medications used, lamotrigine, is both a mood stabilizer and an antidepressant and seems to have a better track record at staving off depression in bipolar patients than the antidepressants do. Please discuss any mood stabilizer in depth with your prescribing physician, and make sure that you understand all of the risks and potential benefits prior to taking it.

Almost all of us experience waves of depression and anxiety in our lifetimes. And some of us are afflicted far too often. There are a wide variety of options that can help support your mood. And the most important of those are not the ones that you put in your mouth. They are talking to someone you care about, getting exercise, basking in the sunshine, getting good sleep, and eating an anti-inflammatory diet. I just saw a 65-year-old patient of mine who is a smart, feisty, and creative world traveller. She is usually actively pursuing her life and too busy to see me, but at this visit, I barely recognized her. Her hair was long, her face sunken, and her eyes cast down. She looked like she was chronically ill. What she was was deeply immersed in grief and depression – for the last 4 months. Her beloved dog of many years had just died and she was roiling in grief and unable to eat. She had a new puppy, but it was annoying and exhausting. She only came in because I insisted on seeing her to refill her blood pressure medication. At that visit, we started SAM-e, 200 milligrams, in the morning. Three days later, she started St. John's wort, 450 milligrams twice daily, and 3 days after that, methyl folic acid at 3 milligrams, with vitamin B_6, methyl B_{12}, and magnesium. I insisted that she walk outside daily. At her following visit 2 weeks later, she came back in with a remarkable turnaround in her symptoms. She was still sad, but crying less. She was getting out of the house and was able to care for her new puppy for the first time in months. I suspect that at our next follow-up, she'll be getting back to her normal self.

We all need help from time to time. I hope that some of these ideas to support your mood connect with your bodywise intuition about what you need and help you have the full, celebratory life that you deserve. As we become bodywise, we can learn to listen to the needs of our bodies and souls

Health Workup for Depression and Anxiety

- Optimal thyroid function: TSH, free T3, free T4
- In a perimenopausal or menopausal woman, hormonal tests can also be helpful: oestradiol, progesterone, testosterone (free and total), and DHEA
- If fatigue or chronic anxiety is present: salivary adrenal testing
- Levels of vitamin B_{12}, folic acid, and homocysteine (an indicator of folic acid metabolism)
- In some cases, especially with a strong family history of depression, genetic testing for methylation defects can help predict useful nutritional treatment (MTHFR A1298C and C677T)

and make choices that allow us to maintain our wholeness, even when we want or need to give to others. If we aren't able to listen to our own needs, or we listen but ignore those needs, we can easily slip into anxiety and depression. Being bodywise means putting our physical and mental well-being first. It is only then that we can be the kind of friend, partner, mother, or contributor to society that we want to be.

CHAPTER 7

Are You Attacking You? Healing Allergies and Autoimmune Conditions

Allergies and Autoimmune Quiz

1. Do you have, or have you had, an irritated skin condition, such as eczema or psoriasis?

1	2	3	4	5
(Never)	(Rarely)	(Sometimes)	(Usually)	(Almost always)

2. Does your skin react to perfumes, lotions, or sunscreens?

1	2	3	4	5
(Never)	(Rarely)	(Sometimes)	(Usually)	(Almost always)

3. Are you allergic to animals, pollens (hay fever), dust, mould, or airborne chemicals, with sneezing, congestion, runny nose, wheezing, or itchy eyes?

1	2	3	4	5
(Never)	(Rarely)	(Sometimes)	(Usually)	(Almost always)

4. Do you react to certain things that you eat or drink (foods, beverages, or medicines) with skin reactions, mouth swelling, stomach pains, nausea, bloating, diarrhoea, constipation, asthma, or altered ability to think?

1	2	3	4	5
(Never)	(Rarely)	(Sometimes)	(Usually)	(Almost always)

5. Do you have asthma or ever need an inhaler for cough or shortness of breath?

1	2	3	4	5
(Never)	(Rarely)	(Sometimes)	(Usually)	(Almost always)

(continued)

Allergies and Autoimmune Quiz (*cont.*)

6. Do you have, or have you ever had, symptoms or test results indicating an autoimmune disease, such as Hashimoto's hypothyroidism, Grave's disease, psoriasis, rheumatoid arthritis, lupus, Crohn's disease, ulcerative colitis, type 1 diabetes, vitiligo, or pernicious anaemia?

1	2	3	4	5
(Never)	(Once in my past)	(2 or more in the past)	(1 currently or 3 or more in the past)	(2 currently or 4 or more in the past)

Add the numbers of your answers.

Your Allergy and Autoimmune score is: _____

If you scored:

6-9: minimal symptoms of allergy/autoimmune issues

10-15: moderate symptoms of allergy/autoimmune issues

16-30: significant symptoms of allergy/autoimmune issues

Our immune systems are like our own Amazon armies – willing and ready to protect us from the dangers of invasion and infection. And when the immune system initially developed to protect us, many thousands of years ago, infections from a variety of organisms (bacteria, worms, parasites, viruses) were common and often deadly. In the Western world, our evolution-honed immune systems now live in disinfected homes rather than the fertile jungles and hot savannahs of our past. And, in general, this is good for us. Sanitation is probably the medical miracle most responsible for our increased life span. The downside is that we now have an army of Amazon warriors on high alert that have fewer fights to occupy them. And this creates new health challenges.

Our overly 'Mr. Clean' environment is one of several causes driving the worldwide epidemic of allergy and autoimmune disease – what I call the body attacking itself – that has been increasing for the last 50 years. Our immune systems, instead of regularly fighting off parasites and bacteria, become overly aggressive with *the wrong targets*. When our immune systems attack benign proteins in our environment (foods, plants, animals, insects, moulds, chemicals, and medications), we call it allergy. When our immune systems attack our own bodies' cells, we call it autoimmune disease.

Women make up 75 per cent of all autoimmune patients in the United States, most probably because our immune systems are slightly more aggressive than men's (I told you we were Amazons). Poignantly, both allergy and autoimmune disease are more likely to become virulent when we are depleted. This is why I often see allergy and autoimmune challenges in women with chronic body depletion. The problems arise when the immune system attacks and overreacts. As a result, we suffer collateral damage, which ranges from a runny nose and sneezing to severe diarrhoea and bleeding intestines to, in rare circumstances, anaphylactic shock, which can be life-threatening.

Megan is a strong and practically minded 33-year-old nurse who came to see me with ongoing, severe skin rashes. During our initial visit, the itching was so intense that she could not stop scratching. She lifted the loose pants she wore to show me weeping, even bleeding, angry red rashes on her shins and similar rashes on both arms. As I do with all of my patients, I asked Megan, 'How did this start? What was happening in your life?' A year and a half prior to seeing me, Megan had accidentally fallen pregnant with a passionate new boyfriend and, despite both their fears of parenthood and a relationship, they were looking for a place to move in together. While making love and trying to open her heart to him, she reached up and discovered a used condom under his pillow – from sex with another woman the day before. In the heavy days that followed, he packed his things and left her – homeless and pregnant. She subsequently had a lonely and painful miscarriage while staying in a friend's basement.

Megan moved to California to begin a new life and found a small home nestled under the redwoods in a beautiful mountainside area. Shortly after her move, a spiritual counsellor recommended that she forgive her ex-partner and reunite 'to work out past life issues that they had together.' Believing that the spiritual counsellor had wisdom greater than hers, she invited her ex-partner to move in with her again, and supported him financially by working night shifts. Within weeks of his moving in, she developed severe allergies, including nasal congestion and sneezing, and then progressed to having asthma symptoms. Her eyes were so itchy that she actually gave herself a corneal abrasion (a scratch on her eyeball) by rubbing them too much and needed to wear an eye patch for several days. Her doctors prescribed steroid eye drops, plus an additional allergy eye drop, several antihistamine tablets, and Flonase – a steroid nasal spray. In addition, she required steroid inhalers to treat her emerging asthma.

One year later, Megan began to have pelvic pain and was diagnosed with pelvic inflammatory disease, a pelvic infection caused by an STD from her unfaithful partner. Sex with him had resulted in a kidney infection as well, and she had needed to take three rounds of very strong antibiotics to treat both infections. She kicked the boyfriend out.

It never ceases to amaze me that often what my patients are experiencing in their outer lives is also happening, physiologically, inside their bodies. Megan's sexual organs were saying 'no' about as loud and clear as they could, to being with this man. She had not one, but two infections of her pelvic area. And when she invited him back into her life, her Amazon immune army went a little nuts – reacting allergically in her eyes, her nose, and her lungs. In bodywise language, her body was communicating about what she couldn't see (her eyes) and whether she could really breathe (her nose and lungs) in this relationship. Megan had poor emotional boundaries in her relationship, and her immune system had poor boundaries in its reactivity – reacting to benign things in the environment allergically. Megan was finally tested by an allergist and found to be allergic to dust mites. She found a new apartment, where she was careful to prevent dust mite exposure. Her asthma and allergy symptoms improved in her new location – free of the cheating boyfriend and the dust mites. However, her skin rashes and itching and scratching continued.

Before I saw Megan, she had three more severe skin infections with high fevers and was treated with three more rounds of antibiotics, two courses of oral steroids, and three steroid shots. In medicine, we use steroids to suppress the immune system in a broad way when it is causing damage to the body – in Megan's case, nasal allergy, asthma, and severe rashes. The steroids temporarily reduce the inflammatory reaction, but do nothing to help with the underlying reasons that the immune system is overreactive.

Our immune systems are intimately connected to our gut bacteria, and when we kill or suppress some gut bacteria with antibiotics and steroids, it allows other unhealthy bacteria and yeast to grow. Our Amazon immune systems are then even further activated, trying to attack and eliminate unhealthy bacteria and yeast growth in the intestines. And in that reactive environment, we are more likely to develop food sensitivities and allergies. Healthy bacteria in the intestines are vital to our health; in fact, we have 10 times as many bacterial cells as human cells! We are an eating, breathing ecosystem with our friends, our intestinal bacteria. In Megan's case, the antibiotics and the steroids had caused disruption of her intestinal bacteria and her Amazon army was on the rampage. Megan was at risk of developing food sensitivity or food allergy, in addition to her other active allergy responses: asthma and hay fever. Megan's intestinal bacteria had been dealt a serious blow in the last 7 months.

When I saw Megan for the first time, we approached her symptoms in a comprehensive way. We began our treatment by asking what her body was trying to tell her. Megan was very clear that the relationship with her ex-boyfriend was harmful to her both emotionally and physically. I asked her if she had had similar problems with other people in her life, and she recognized that she had had difficulty with setting boundaries – certainly with the ex-boyfriend – but also with friends and colleagues on an ongoing basis. She realized that listening to her spiritual counsellor's advice over her own body intuition had clearly been a mistake.

In order to heal, Megan acknowledged that she needed to set healthy boundaries around relationships. She also needed to identify what her body was currently reacting to and avoid it. We stopped all topical prescription medications and lotions that had multiple chemicals in them (in case she was reacting to them) and had her use only coconut oil or olive oil and beeswax ointments. We also tested her for food allergies and sensitivities.

Megan had improved a little by our second visit, but continued to have milder arm and leg rashes. The testing revealed no actual food allergies, but she did have some sensitivity to citrus and eggs – both of which she stopped eating. We started her on natural anti-inflammatory foods and supplements: flaxseed oil and evening primrose oil, and lots of brightly coloured fruits and vegetables. (The colour in fruits and vegetables is actually the anti-oxidant that is anti-inflammatory.) We took a look at her gut bacterial profile, and, not surprisingly given all of the antibiotics she had taken, her gut was very low in healthy bacteria and had inflammation present; we treated this with high-dose probiotics (at least 100 billion CFU or colony forming units), glutamine (a benign amino acid that reduces gut inflammation), and prebiotics – soluble fibres that help the healthy bacteria grow. And because we can't get all the healthy gut bacteria we need from supplements, I encouraged her to eat fermented foods as well – a natural source of healthy bacteria (sauerkraut, tempeh, kefir, kombucha, and kimchee, to name a few).

Megan had a dramatic improvement in her rash with all of the above treatments, and when I last saw her, she had just a small remaining rash on one arm that we treated with a topical ointment. I expect her to be fully cured at our next appointment. And for Megan, becoming bodywise – listening to her body's signals – was the key to her getting well. She is now starting to date again, but is being careful to listen to the intelligence from the front line of her body as she chooses her next partner – so the Amazons don't go on the warpath again.

One of the concepts that is important to understand is that our immune systems can be extremely specific, reacting, say, to ragweed pollen but not to oak tree pollen. At the same time, the immune system has a general volume control. A person who has asthma, an allergic response of the bronchial tubes and lungs, may have a worsening of her asthma symptoms when she is eating a food she is allergic to and living in an environment where she is sensitive to pollens and moulds. The cumulative effect of exposure to multiple allergens increases the strength – and inflammatory damage – of the overall allergic immune response. In this way, multiple rounds of antibiotics can disrupt the gut bacteria, predispose one to develop a food sensitivity or allergy, and then increase the overall vigorousness of the allergic immune response.

Here is an example of what I'm talking about. Trevor is an adorable, active 8-year-old boy in my practice. Trevor had mild asthmatic reactions as a baby and toddler when he had colds or flus. Unfortunately, he developed ear infections at ages 3 and 4, and had six rounds of antibiotics. By the time I saw him, he had also developed eczema, an allergic skin rash, and his asthma had worsened to require daily treatment. I referred Trevor to an allergist who diagnosed him as being allergic to dust mites, mould, and cow dairy. His mum and I set about cleaning up his environment to minimize dust mites and mould and took him off of all dairy products. With these allergens absent in his environment, his immune system was able to settle, and his eczema cleared. He no longer required daily asthma treatments and used his inhalers just when he was getting ill. Next, we set about restoring his gut bacteria from the damage the antibiotics had caused, so that he wasn't vulnerable to developing more allergies, using glutamine, prebiotics, probiotics, and fermented foods, as we did with Megan.

Understanding Autoimmune Disease

Unfortunately, 1 out of 12 women in the United States will have autoimmune disease in her lifetime. The most common autoimmune disease, Hashimoto's thyroiditis, which causes low thyroid function, is a woman's disease 90 per cent of the time. Because autoimmune disease and allergy both stem from an overreactive (and inappropriately reactive) immune response, their prevention and natural treatment are very similar.

As you can see in the list (opposite), the symptoms of autoimmune disease are quite diverse: joint pain, abdominal pain and bloody diarrhoea, skin rashes, or dry eyes and mouth, to name a few. But most of the autoimmune diseases are connected in that sufferers are almost inevitably exhausted, and even flulike, with low energy and body aches.

Leila was a tired, sad, but motivated woman who arrived in my office inspired by having seen a recent educational summit about autoimmune disease. Like many patients with autoimmune disease, Leila's illness started with severe physical stress. She was a self-described type-A person and a successful businesswoman who was well prior to being struck down with severe bacterial meningitis, 25 years earlier. She recovered from the meningitis, but began what was to be a long and debilitating journey with systemic lupus. Leila had small children at the time of her diagnosis and was living with a husband who was alcoholic and emotionally abusive. As you might imagine, this all contributed to her symptoms.

Leila has been seen and treated at some of the best medical institutions in the world, but despite an enormous number of treatments, she has been 90 per cent bedridden with a combination of lupus, chronic fatigue, insomnia, chronic migraines, and ongoing bloating and constipation. Both her mother and her daughter have subsequently also been diagnosed with lupus, and her daughter has an additional autoimmune disease as well. Leila also suffered from allergies to dust mites, trees, and grasses. She is a classic example of someone with an immune system on fire.

Over the past few months, Leila had stopped eating gluten and dairy and limited her diet to only organic foods with no GMOs (genetically modified organisms). She had also started a number of vitamins including vitamin D_3, magnesium, B-complex, zinc, fish oil, vitamin B_{12}, and glutathione. When I first saw her in my clinic, I was particularly concerned about nutrition. Leila was taking 29 medications, including a chemotherapy medication

Types of Autoimmune Disease

Addison's disease: adrenal hormone insufficiency

Coeliac disease: a reaction to gluten (found in wheat, rye, and barley) that causes damage to the lining of the small intestine

Graves' disease: overactive thyroid gland

Hashimoto's thyroiditis: underactive thyroid gland

Inflammatory bowel diseases (IBD): a group of inflammatory diseases of the colon and small intestine, including Crohn's disease and ulcerative colitis

Pernicious anaemia: reduced number of red blood cells caused by inability to absorb vitamin B_{12}

Psoriasis: a skin condition that causes redness and irritation as well as thick, flaky, silver-white patches

Reactive arthritis: inflammation of joints, urethra, and eyes; may cause sores on the skin and mucous membranes

Rheumatoid arthritis: inflammation of joints and surrounding tissues

Scleroderma: a connective tissue disease that causes changes in skin, blood

vessels, muscles, and internal organs

Sjögren's syndrome: destroys the glands that produce tears and saliva, causing dry eyes and mouth; may affect kidneys and lungs

Systemic lupus erythematosus: affects skin, joints, kidneys, brain, and other organs

Type 1 diabetes: destruction of insulin-producing cells in the pancreas

Vitiligo: white patches on the skin caused by loss of pigment

used for autoimmune disease, and a number of other medications that were known to reduce B vitamin and magnesium levels in the body. I ordered a comprehensive stool test to examine her GI flora, food allergy and food sensitivity testing, and a deep nutritional test.

Leila also suffered from insomnia and had been diagnosed with obstructive sleep apnoea many years before, but was not using her CPAP (continuous positive airway pressure) machine because it dried out her mouth at night. I encouraged her to find a better-fitting CPAP mask and to use it, as healing sleep was essential to treating her autoimmune condition.

On her return visit, she also let me know about severe balance problems she was having and some significant issues with her short-term memory. A laboratory blood test showed that she had no food allergies and only had a very mild food sensitivity to bananas. Because of her ongoing fatigue, I also tested her MTHFR genetic profile (see Chapter 6), and two of her four genes were abnormal. Because of this, we started her on activated methyl folic acid, B_{12}, B_6, and magnesium, to assist with energy and her MTHFR deficits. Nutritional testing showed her to be functionally deficient in all of the B vitamins and all of the fat-soluble vitamins as well. She had evidence of excessive oxidation (a cause of inflammation) in her body and had a deficit of antioxidants (vitamins A, E, K, and C) to balance this. Her stool testing showed that she had very poor fat-digestion ability, which would impair the absorption of vitamins A, D, E, and K – important antioxidants. (These tests would usually be done by a complementary health practitioner in the UK). Leila had evidence of poor detoxification and low glutathione (an important antioxidant and detoxifier). With all of these issues, it was no wonder that she felt so ill.

Leila had already been taking supplemental glutathione, but we tripled her dose. Glutathione, when taken by mouth, is absorbed on a limited basis. Some experts recommend giving the precursors to glutathione: N-acetyl cysteine, glutamine and glycine. Another option with preliminary research showing increased abortion into the blood, is micronized glutathione – glutathione in microscopic bubbles that deliver it through the intestinal lining. We added an antioxidant supplement and a higher-quality fish oil that also contained the omega-6 GLA (gamma linolenic acid). I have found that adding GLA to the omega-3s is useful for many of my patients with inflammatory disorders, such as eczema or even rosacea. Common sources of GLA are evening primrose, borage, or blackcurrant seed oil.

Stool testing had also shown an overgrowth of unfriendly bacteria and insufficient healthy good bacteria. We started a digestive enzyme before meals to assist with her poor fat digestion. And we treated her bacterial overgrowth with a broad antibacterial herbal supplement, followed by a potent probiotic for several months. Because of her mild reaction to banana, we had her avoid banana for several months during this healing process.

At our next visit, Leila was using her CPAP and felt less fatigued. She was also able to take most of her supplements, and was feeling a slow improvement in her lupus symptoms. Also, she had significantly less gas and bloating after taking the herbs for bacterial overgrowth. She had more energy and fewer headaches.

We continued everything she was taking, and when I saw Leila 4 months later, I barely recognized her. She had had an almost miraculous reversal of her lupus symptoms and her chronic fatigue and was active for most of the day. She felt well enough to drive across the country to go on holiday with her children for the first time. Her balance issues have resolved and she only has rare migraines. She is actively weaning off many of her medications, with the support of her doctor.

Leila's treatment may seem complex, because her illnesses were complex, but the steps that I helped Leila take are the same ones I use with all of my patients with significant allergies and autoimmune disease. These are:

1. Reduce stress and support normal adrenal function.
2. Reduce inflammation in your body with foods and supplements.
3. Identify any allergic reactions you might have.
4. Take steps to avoid what you react to (including people).
5. Test your gut.
6. Use medications when you need them.

Reduce Stress and Support Normal Adrenal Function

Like Megan or Leila above, most of my patients with autoimmune disease tell me a story of illness, extreme stress, or loss that occurred with the first symptoms of their autoimmune disease. It is well-established that ongoing stress substantially affects immune function and makes allergy and autoimmune reactions flare for the first time. And increased stress can exacerbate an autoimmune disorder that had been under control. In a fascinating study, patients with asthma and rheumatoid arthritis were asked to write in a journal about stressful experiences in their lives. After doing so for 4 months, there were substantial, measurable improvements in both the asthma and the rheumatoid arthritis symptoms.[1] Simply writing about life stress helps to get it out there, so to speak, rather than keeping it inside where it inflames the immune system.

If stress can cause allergy and autoimmune symptoms, then stress reduction can relieve those symptoms. As we discussed in the last chapter, any meditation or prayer activity can substantially reduce our stress markers. Gentle exercise can be extremely helpful, too, especially yoga, tai chi, or qigong. Autoimmune patients also frequently have chronic pain, and exercise is essential for keeping the pain contained. We discussed adrenal support in Chapter 3, including reducing caffeine and taking B vitamins, as needed. And the most anti-inflammatory behaviour we can benefit from is deep sleep, so getting enough sleep and making sure your sleep is of good quality (like Leila did by wearing her CPAP mask) is essential.

Reduce Inflammation in Your Body

In allergy and autoimmune disease, inflammation is caused by an overactive immune response. We can counteract the damage wrought by the immune system by eating an anti-inflammatory diet, rich in brightly coloured fruits and vegetables, nuts, and fish. You may also want to take anti-inflammatory supplements, such as curcumin, green tea, ginger, bromelain, boswellia (Frankincense), or vitamin D. There are a variety of supplements on the market that combine these powerful anti-inflammatories; these are particularly helpful in patients with arthritis and inflammatory bowel disease, but can be useful for any allergy or autoimmune reaction. I would also recommend a high-quality fish oil omega-3 supplement with at least 1,000 milligrams of EPA and 500 milligrams of DHA. In addition, I have seen some very positive responses to adding the omega-6, GLA, to omega-3 therapy, at 600 milligrams one to two times daily. GLA acts through a different enzyme chain to increase DGLA, which has an anti-inflammatory effect. In someone with significant airborne allergies with a runny nose and sneezing, I have also had good success with the anti-inflammatory product isoquercitrin, which is a more bioavailable form of quercetin. Quercetin is a flavonoid derived from the pigments of red fruits, like apples or berries, and is anti-inflammatory, but also has antihistamine properties. It can be used at the recommended dose twice daily to reduce itchy eyes and runny nose, much like a prescription antihistamine, but with fewer side effects (no dry mouth, reduced cardiovascular risk, and improved immune function).

Identify Any Allergic Reactions You Might Have

Identifying the source of someone's immune reactivity helps us limit that exposure. Avoiding exposure, when possible, is much easier on the body than treating the symptoms with immune suppressants, such as steroids. For environmental allergies, you can request that your doctor order blood (IgE) or skin allergy testing, though skin allergy testing is more accurate for airborne allergens (pollen, animals, dust mites, mould). Food allergies can also be diagnosed through skin prick testing at an allergist's office. Keep in mind that food allergy testing, which measures IgE levels of reaction against foods, is not entirely accurate. And food sensitivity testing, even less so! This is why many doctors don't use food sensitivity testing. I am picky about which labs I use for food sensitivity, as some of them give such positive results for seemingly unrelated and nonallergenic foods, that I find them impossible to use clinically. The gold standard for food sensitivity, and even food allergy, is the elimination and challenge diet. In its classic form, you remove the five most allergenic foods – cow dairy, soy, eggs, peanuts, and gluten – for 2 weeks. Then, you add each one of them back in for 3 days, and remove it again, noting any changes in symptoms. This takes some significant discipline, but it is a hugely valuable exercise! But if you, like Megan above, are allergic to something *not* included in one of those food groups (in her case, citrus), you won't discover it. This is the primary reason that I test for food allergy and sensitivity; it allows me to do a more focused examination of what this particular patient's body is responding to. I give instructions on the elimination and challenge diet in the BodyWise 28-Day Plan at the end of the book.

Now, can someone be negative on both food allergy and food sensitivity testing and still react to a food? Yes! This is an area in which to really use your bodywise listening to discern what works and doesn't work for your body. My patients are usually remarkably accurate about what they *think* they are reacting to; it is often what they are actually reacting to. You might not always *like* the answer, especially if it means giving up something that you love, but when you really pay attention to what you're eating and how your body responds, you'll be amazed by how quickly you're able to identify your triggers. If you know that eating aubergine makes you feel bad, don't eat it! Your body is more finely tuned than a blood test.

If you have severe autoimmune disease and are not improving, you may want to consider going on an autoimmune diet, which avoids foods that are potentially the most inflammatory to your immune system. These include all dairy, all gluten, all soy, eggs, peanuts, legumes, tree nuts, and all grains. You ask, reasonably, 'What the hell am I supposed to eat?' And my answer is meat, fish, vegetables and fruit, along with quinoa, wild rice, and amaranth (which are not actually grains). That is the autoimmune diet. If you improve rapidly on it, you can slowly introduce each of the eliminated foods as we treat your gut and normalize your immune response.

Because of the gluten-free craze, I want to specifically address gluten as a food group. Gluten is the protein within several grains: wheat (including spelt, farro, semolina, kamut, and other wheat forms), rye, barley, and triticale. Severe gluten allergy causes severe disease, referred to as coeliac disease. This can be diagnosed by a blood test at a regular lab, which is pretty accurate, but occasionally misses cases. It is also diagnosed through biopsies of the intestine, as gluten allergy wreaks so much damage on the endothelial cells that line the intestines. Coeliac disease is serious, and people with this condition need to religiously avoid gluten in all forms.

There are certainly people who are gluten sensitive, like my patient who, after 30 years, got rid of chronic migraines by going off gluten. Gluten-sensitive people can have worsened rashes or allergy symptoms, abdominal pain, diarrhoea or constipation, or fatigue when they eat gluten. The best way to find out if you are sensitive is to stop gluten for 2 to 4 weeks, and then add it back in. How do you feel? As with many foods, some people can eat a little gluten and be fine. But a loaf of French bread with pasta alfredo with seitan (wheat gluten) meatballs will push them over the edge of the gluten cliff. One health condition that drives me to ask people to try going off gluten for a period of time, regardless of their testing, is Hashimoto's hypothyroidism, which has a clear antibody overlap with gluten. I have had to readjust my patients' thyroid medication levels when they've gone off gluten because the autoimmune attack recedes a bit and the thyroid gland 'wakes up' and starts functioning again.

I do not think gluten is evil or that avoiding gluten is a panacea for treating all illnesses. I do think that most of us evolved to be able to eat a variety of foods, including wheat. I also think that we've done some funny things with our wheat grains in the United States, and I continue to hear stories from my gluten-sensitive patients about how they can eat European bread, no problem. Some wheat may be more allergenic than others. If you have coeliac disease, avoid gluten at all costs. If you are gluten-sensitive, pay attention to your body, and avoid it if it makes your symptoms worse. If after taking gluten out of your diet for several weeks and adding it back in, you feel no different, it is fine to eat gluten. In fact, gluten is a higher-protein grain than its common substitute – rice. Stopping gluten to eat more rice will result in your eating more carbohydrates, less protein, and fewer vitamins, as rice is not a very nutritious grain. Other wheat substitutes, such as quinoa, amaranth, or millet, are healthier choices.

Identifying allergies and sensitivities of all kinds is essential to improving allergy and autoimmune disease by treating the source of the symptoms, the allergen itself.

Take Steps to Avoid What You React To

Removing an autoimmune or allergic trigger from your life can be a challenge, but I promise you that I have seen some miraculous improvements in symptoms when my patients are able to avoid or limit their allergen triggers. The kind of health and vitality that are available to you when your body is not in a chronic immune response is remarkable. You can go from pain and flulike symptoms to really feeling like yourself again. Avoiding foods that you are truly allergic to, or have strong negative reactions to, is essential, but often takes willpower. I find that most of my patients get into the groove of their new allergen-free diets in about a month, as it takes time to create new patterns of shopping and cooking. Note that if you are simply sensitive to a food, rather than allergic, you may be able to eat it again after doing a gut-healing regime (below).

For airborne allergies, there are other strategies. If dust mites are an issue, you will want dust covers for your pillows and mattress, available online and at many stores that carry products for the bedroom. An in-room HEPA (high-efficiency particulate air) filter and HEPA-filter vacuum cleaner can reduce airborne allergens, such as pollen and animal dander. If you suffer from significant allergies or asthma and suspect mould in your home, it may be worth the investment to have a professional come in and test for mould spores. There are even inexpensive mould-culture kits that you can order online for this purpose and check it out yourself. You'll find guidance for avoiding dust mites and other allergens in Appendix A. One of the harder situations in my clinic is the allergic patient who is allergic to her beloved dog or cat. I usually argue for keeping Fido or Fifi out of the bedroom, where you spend most of your time at home, and using a HEPA air filter in the bedroom.

Test Your Gut

Balancing the gut can be the fundamental stepping-stone for reversing allergy and autoimmune disease. Find a practitioner who can order a stool test that describes stool function and identifies stool bacterial populations in detail. This is typically a holistic or complementary health practitioner, and Appendix B lists resources for finding someone in your area. That practitioner will help eliminate gut infections (parasites, yeast, or bacterial overgrowth, for example); eliminate food allergens from your diet; restore your normal gut bacteria (with prebiotics, probiotics, and fermented foods); and reduce gut inflammation (with compounds such as fish oil, turmeric,

Health Workup for Allergies and Autoimmune Conditions

- For environmental allergies causing sneezing, congestion, itchy eyes, or asthma, ideally see an allergist for skin testing for allergies to trees and grasses in your area, animals, mould, and dust mites or other insects. An IgE blood test, widely available at all labs, for all these is a secondary possibility – not as accurate, but better than no testing.

- For food allergies, both skin testing (make sure all relevant foods are included) and blood testing (for IgE) are equally valid and equally not entirely reliable. Still, they can point you in the right direction.

- Food sensitivity testing may be useful if all the above testing is negative. It is even less reliable than food allergy testing, so I use it as a guide for the best food test – an elimination diet. A guide to an elimination diet is included in the 28-day plan on page 221. You will probably need an integrative physician or naturopath to obtain this testing (see Appendix B).

- C-reactive protein (CRP): to look for chronic inflammation, which may indicate an underlying medical disorder, including active autoimmune disease.

- Arthritis panel – if significant inflammatory joint pain is the issue – RF (rheumatoid factor) and ANA (antinuclear antigen). If either of these is elevated, other clarifying tests should be ordered by your doctor or rheumatologist.

- Thyroid function, as it can undermine immune function: TSH, free T3, free T4, and anti-TPO antibodies (the antibody test for Hashimoto's hypothyroidism).

- 25-hydroxy vitamin D (low levels of vitamin D double the risk for autoimmune disease, and in a patient with autoimmune disease, the level should be greater than 40 ng/ml).

- Salivary adrenal testing, if fatigue is an issue. This is typically performed by a holistic or naturopathic doctor, or acupuncturist, or can be accessed at online labs.

- Comprehensive stool testing: This cannot be done by regular labs, as they do not test for the species of normal bacteria in the intestine. It is much easier to obtain this testing from a holistic doctor or naturopath (see Appendix B).

DGL, or deglycyrrhizinated liquorice, glutamine, and aloe). If it is not possible to see an integrative practitioner and do stool testing, it's still helpful to keep your gut healthy by eating lots of fruits and vegetables (healthy fibre feeds the gut bacteria and is an anti-inflammatory), eating fermented foods (yogurt, kefir, sauerkraut, kimchee, kombucha, tempeh, miso), and taking a probiotic, preferably a high-potency one (see Appendix A).

Use Medications When You Need Them

The point of the recommendations above for healing allergy and auto-immune disease is to keep you from needing medication or help to limit the toxic medications that you have to take. However, medication plays a role in the treatment of allergy and autoimmune disease. When my patients with seasonal allergies are miserable with sneezing and runny noses, I encourage them to use a steroid nasal spray. It can cause nosebleeds, but it is relatively benign and can be enormously helpful with symptoms. Antihistamines such as loratadine, fexofenadine, or cetirizine can also be helpful, as are allergy eye drops. In patients with severe airborne allergies, sometimes allergy shots, which reduce the immune response by giving small doses of the aller-gen over time, can be remarkably effective.

The use of medications for asthma needs its own discussion, as those medications can sometimes be lifesaving. With my asthma patients, I use the above interventions to try to reduce their reliance on medications, but I would be the first one to encourage regular use of steroid inhalers when they have regular symptoms of asthma. In some patients, like Megan, I'm able to keep their asthma symptoms controlled by natural means, and they're able to stop their steroid inhalers. However, in many patients, we might start steroid inhalers to prevent a severe asthma exacerbation or use them regu-larly, if symptoms are ongoing. None of the natural interventions is harmful to your asthma management, but I would strongly urge you to discuss any possible changes in asthma medication with your practitioner.

If you suffer from autoimmune disease, medication treatment is com-plex. In part, this is because the medications that we currently have to alter and calm the immune response have a tremendous number of side effects and long-term risks. In certain situations, those risks are worth it as they stabilize an otherwise potentially fatal disease, such as severely activated inflammatory bowel disease or severely debilitating systemic arthritis or lupus. Long-term use of disease-modifying medications should always be discussed with your rheumatologist or GP prior to change. Your holistic doctor and your specialist have the same goal: that your disease is controlled and that any permanent damage to your joints or organs is averted. Some-times this means staying on your disease-modifying medication for your own health. I've always worked with my patients' specialists and, together, we do not recommend reducing or changing medications until the lab tests and physical symptoms that we use to monitor the disease are improved.

Using the bodywise principles, I have had great success in helping my patients with allergies and autoimmune disease improve their symptoms. And when they improve their symptoms and immune reactivity, they feel more vibrant and able. And we can avoid or decrease their dangerous medications. Now that's being bodywise.

PART THREE

Using Your Body Wisdom to Heal Your Life

Our lifestyle choices are responsible for fully 88 per cent of the illnesses that drive people to the doctor. How we eat, move, sleep, love, and find a sense of purpose determines *most* of our wellness. The good news is that an enormous percentage of what ails us can be prevented or cured by becoming more bodywise and acting in accordance with our own intuition and well-being. While I have said that everyone's body is different, there are some fundamental things that all people need – and that even the arguing experts can agree upon. Everyone, regardless of gender, race, class, or country, needs nutritious food, restful sleep, physical activity to stay strong and fit, love and community, and a sense of purpose for being on planet earth. These fundamentals of health are the treatment and cure for chronic body depletion. In this part of the book, you will learn how to apply these fundamentals to your specific needs. These principles can support you to live a life that your body will love.

CHAPTER 8

Eat: Weight Gain, Weight Loss, and Nourishing Your Body

Lakshmi is a 55-year-old patient of mine who weighs 190 pounds and is 5 feet 4 inches tall. She cycles 20 to 40 miles three times a week, does yoga, and eats healthy food.

Katie is a 30-year-old patient of mine who weighs 125 pounds and is 5 feet 9 inches tall. She exercises daily for 60 minutes, doing aerobics classes or running 6 miles. Her diet is vegan and gluten-free.

Lakshmi has perfect blood pressure and cholesterol, a happy marriage and kids, a great sex life, and an almost perfect in-depth nutritional analysis. Lakshmi struggles to lose weight despite much effort to do so, as did her mum after menopause, but she is otherwise happy with her body.

Katie has very low blood pressure and hypoglycaemia. Her cholesterol is too low, and she has severely deficient nutrition according to in-depth testing. Katie complains of low libido, fatigue, and joint pain. Katie struggles with anorexia and hates her body.

Both of these patients need my help, but Lakshmi, who is severely overweight by medical standards, is otherwise very healthy – in mind, body, and soul. She is a bodywise woman who simply has a difficult time losing weight and needs gentle guidance and strategy. Katie, on the other hand, may be thin, but is really the opposite of bodywise. She ignores, and at this point can't even feel, her body's hunger signals. She suffers from anxiety and depression, and her intense exercise programme actually exacerbates her severe adrenal dysfunction. She is chronically tired, but ignores that signal as she continues to push herself, which results in further injuries and illness.

She even has an altered visual perception of her body – seeing someone who is fat in the mirror, despite the fact that she looks more like a victim of starvation. Katie rules her body with derision and deprivation, ignoring what her body is screaming at her to do: Rest. Sleep. Eat.

Both Lakshmi and Katie struggle to be women who feel good in their bodies in a culture that is obsessed with what women look like on the outside, rather than how they feel on the inside. Making decisions about what to eat multiple times a day can be a tricky business in modern culture. All women are different, and all of us have different nutritional needs in different life stages. Pregnant women famously have cravings, and often this is their bodies telling them what they need. I have been vegetarian, vegan, and fishetarian (vegetarian plus fish) for more than 30 years. But when I was pregnant with my son in my late twenties, I remember driving by a billboard for a local steak house with a giant, steaming, juicy steak on it. I literally slowed my car to gaze at the steak longingly, thinking, 'Wow, that looks *really* good.' My body was clearly telling me what it wanted and needed – more protein and iron – regardless of my preferences. It still does. And I try my best to listen.

Given the confusing world of competing food recommendations, the pressure to look a certain way, and the intense marketing of foods that are bad for us, it is not a simple feat to sense one's own intuition. Add to that the intensely addictive quality of food – especially sugar and processed foods – and it can be a challenge to hear what your body *really* wants. The first part of becoming bodywise around food choices is to honour your own intuition above any external voice in your head – including me – about what you should eat.

You can use the bodywise tools to help discern what your body needs

Here is how you can use the bodywise method to help you out. Next time you're ready to eat, take a few deep belly breaths. Close your eyes and sink attention into your body, using the body feelings exercise (see page 34) to help you locate where your hunger is and what it feels like. When you gently consider the feeling of hunger, do any emotions arise? If the emotion is 'I am lightheaded and going to pass out if I don't have a snack,' perhaps it is time for a snack. If the emotion is, 'I'm _____' (fill in the blank: bored, angry, sad, scared, anxious), you may want to take a minute to consider your food choice. Remember that emotional or addictive eating requires that you eat whatever you are craving immediately. Just taking a moment to consider what your body is actually saying can save you from the tub of Häagen-Dazs.

and wants and what is habitual, emotional, or addictive eating. For some women, the first challenge is to actually feel and recognize hunger. Equally important is the ability to recognize and experience fullness.

When you really stop to listen to your body's cues, you may find that you're not actually hungry at all. Most of us, myself included, use food as a reward from time to time; we also eat when we're in a bad mood, upset, bored, and for all kinds of reasons beyond true hunger. Waiting to eat until you're actually hungry is a great skill and a real part of being bodywise, and being aware of the different cues that make you reach for a snack is the first step in shifting your habits away from eating and on to other experiences that can fulfil you. I do want to point out that if you are fatigued, and especially if you have adrenal fatigue, eating small healthy meals regularly is helpful in maintaining your energy. If you can't yet perceive your own hunger, you will still need to eat a healthy snack every 2 to 3 hours to maintain your blood sugar.

Indulging the daily craving for a bag of cookies is a different story, but we all need feel-good rewards now and then. It's only human. When I try to help my patients stop smoking, drinking, or overeating, I often help them to strategize new 'treats' that will be less destructive. Non-food treats can include a hot bath, going outside for a walk/run, putting on loud music that you love and dancing, calling your best friend, reading a book, watching a show you love, or having great sex. All very healthy. Lots of possibilities. And then, when you're actually hungry from your dancing, walking, talking, bathing, or sex activity, you can get some food.

There are some food cravings that are physiological. For example, when I'm sleep deprived (and as a doctor and mother of twins, I have had a lot of practice at this), I crave sugar. But what I've learned is that my tired body is telling me, 'Get me some quick energy here, I'm dying. . . .' And what I really need is a nap. And sometimes, honestly, I crave kale, especially after a long day of work when my body needs sustenance. I know, I'm a geek. But when I really listen, my body tells me it wants all those killer vitamins and minerals. Which is what I tell myself when I crave coffee – all those good antioxidants. . . .

Sometimes, we need food alternatives. If you are really going to lay off the potato crisps, you may need a replacement. For starters, don't keep your 'food crack' in the house. That's not to say that I believe you should never snack; my advice, though, is to find healthy substitutes that will fulfil your cravings without breaking the calorific and nutritional banks. If crunchy/salty is your thing, consider baked nori seaweed with sesame oil and salt (I admit to being fully addicted to this), kale crisps, or popcorn – just don't eat a gallon of it. If your thing is sweet, consider full-fat plain yogurt with healthy sweetener and fruit (see healthy sweeteners on page 151). You can even add unsweetened chocolate powder to full-fat plain Greek yogurt with sweetener, and it tastes like pudding. And – you're going to think I'm nuts – but pureed avocado with chocolate powder and sweetener also really tastes like chocolate pudding. I swear. Not a chocolate girl? Consider plain whipped cream with vanilla and sweetener – it's not calorie-free, but if it's organic cream, your cholesterol is reasonably good, and you use no sweetener or a low-calorie one, it's surprisingly not that bad for you. And, of course, you could add chocolate to it. I've included a recipe for Raw Cacao Balls in Appendix A – not particularly calorie-free, but *very* good for you.

Now, it's important to note that food addiction is a real thing, especially in the case of processed snack foods, fast food, and sugar, in general. These foods actually set up a dopamine response in your brain that puts you into painful *withdrawal* when you stop eating them – causing irritability, anxiety, and intense craving. If this sounds familiar to you, you probably have a real food addiction. And food addiction, like any addiction, can be difficult to break. If it is a specific food that you crave (sugar, soft drinks, and crisps are the most common in my practice), you are probably going to need to stop eating it entirely. It will be difficult for 1 to 2 weeks, as you 'withdraw' from the cravings, but then your brain will adjust, and the cravings will ease. As long as you don't eat it. Just like stopping smoking, choose a time to stop eating your addictive food that is fortuitous – you're busy doing something else you love, your kids are gone to summer camp, the knives have been removed from the house – whatever works. Set a date. Get that shit out of your home. Tell everybody what you're doing and get their support. And stop eating it. You can do this. And if you need support, there are many resources for people with food addictions, from Food Addicts Anonymous to Overeaters Anonymous.

Most important, be kind to yourself. So, if you promised not to eat potato crisps, and in the process of making the stinking kale crisps, you burned them and in frustration drove to 7-Eleven to get the potato crisps, relax. Take a breath. We are human. We err. A lot. And we pick ourselves up and move on. One less potato crisp at a time.

In my practice, I hear about so many food fad diets that restrict one thing or another that sometimes it makes my head spin. 'Dr Rachel, I'm a raw, gluten-free vegan' or 'Dr Rachel, I eat the Zone diet, with a Paleo twist' or 'I'm on a low-glycaemic, vegan plus wild meat diet.' Sometimes, it's actually easier to ask what people *do* eat than what they don't, like my patient who *only* eats courgettes and turkey – but that's another story. And the truth is that everyone needs something a little different, and needs different

BodyWise Eating

- Foods grown or raised without pesticides, hormones, or antibiotics
- Lots of fruits and vegetables
- Beans, legumes, nuts, and seeds as part of our protein requirements
- Good fats like olives and olive oil, nuts and seeds, avocados, and coconut
- Cold-water fish (that is sustainable and low in mercury) and some lean meat (preferably organic and grass-fed)
- Whole grains, if your body likes them
- Organic dairy products, if your body likes them
- Limited natural sweets or sweeteners

things at different seasons of life. There is no perfect permanent eating plan for everyone. That said, smart nutritional experts agree on about 90 per cent of their recommendations. Based on what we actually know from modern nutritional science and evolutionary medicine, ideally we all should eat as outlined in the box above.

When we eat this way, we greatly reduce our risk of heart disease, stroke, cancer, diabetes, autoimmune disease, depression, and obesity – just about everything that makes people sick.

For all of the connotations it has – food is love, food is comfort, and food is pleasure and reward and celebration – food is actually medicine, literally. Everything you put into your mouth has complex biochemical messages for the body. We can heal ourselves with what we eat. And becoming bodywise about what your body wants to eat can save your life.

When trying to navigate the confusing world of food, I find it useful to consider what the human body adapted to eating over the past 10,000 years of our evolution. Food was difficult to come by and required effort to hunt or to gather. Our bodies were honed to eat much less and to work hard to get it. Certain nutrients were essential for our physiology but not always easy to come by in nature, such as concentrated sweets, salt, and fat. Being genetically brilliant, we evolved to crave sugar, salt, and fat. Meat was a rare but very valuable part of our food supply in most cultures. And the great majority of humans were lean, surviving on far fewer calories than people in developed countries consume today.

In contrast, today a small number of multinational corporations control our entire food system. The most common foods eaten in the United States are wheat flour, dairy products, and potatoes, and it's a similar picture in the UK. Unfortunately, most of those potatoes are consumed as French fries. One-quarter of the US population visits a fast-food restaurant daily.[1] The volume of the food we consume has gone up substantially over the past 50 years. Which is one of the reasons that we have the highest rate of obesity in human history. More than one-third of US adults are obese.[2] One in three people born in the year 2000 will develop diabetes, largely as a consequence of being overweight. The current generation will be the first ever to live shorter lives than their parents. This is a sad statement about our values.

There has also been a tremendous loss of diversity in the foods we eat. A large part of the diet in the United States is based on processed foods that combine salt, sweet, and fat in a carefully calculated balance that appeals to our tastebuds and creates addictive cravings. Seventy per cent of processed foods are genetically modified. There is a growing organic food movement in the United States, but it is still the case that the majority of food production uses pesticides for crop production, hormones in animal factory farming, and antibiotics in animal feed to increase animal fat deposition (and produce tender meat). The impact of this massive use of antibiotics is actually terrifying. The broad exposure to antibiotics in our world is creating superbugs – bacteria that have become resistant to any existing antibiotic treatments – at lightning speed. And as discussed, antibiotics in our food supply are further destroying our very important intestinal bacteria that protect us from allergy and disease.

A recent sampling of umbilical cord blood in the United States revealed that more than 200 industrial chemicals were present on average. Of the 287 chemicals detected, 180 cause cancer in humans or animals, 217 are toxic to the brain and nervous system, and 208 cause birth defects or abnormal development in animal tests.[3] And we wonder why we have skyrocketing rates of attention deficit disorder and learning disorders in our children! We have been conducting the biggest experiment on industrialized food and toxic exposure that has ever been seen in human history.

So what can we do? Some of the bright news is that consuming an organic diet for 1 week significantly reduces pesticide exposure, by 89 per cent, compared to a conventional diet.[4] Probably the biggest exposure that we get to pesticides is from the meat and milk of animals who have been fed grain grown with pesticides. Pesticides are fat-soluble, and thus stay in the fat and meat of the animals until they are slaughtered for food, or the pesticides are released into their milk supply. Simply buying organic milk and meat, or limiting meat intake, can make a substantial difference to your pesticide exposure. And although organic milk and meat are more widely available than in the past 25 years, they are still expensive. If you're deciding where to invest your food pounds, splurge on the organic apples and organic meat and milk and buy the regular avocados and corn (which are lower in pesticides). And make up the difference in your food bill by limiting your meat intake, preferring the healthy and more affordable protein sources of beans, grains, and nuts. You will be healthier overall and will also substantially reduce your pesticide exposure. This list from the Environmental Working Group has been very useful for me and my patients.[5]

HIGHEST PESTICIDE CONTENT (LISTED WORST TO BEST)	LOWEST IN PESTICIDES (LISTED BEST TO WORST)
Apples	Avocados
Peaches	Sweet corn
Nectarines	Pineapples
Strawberries	Cabbage
Grapes	Garden peas (frozen)
Celery	Onions
Spinach	Asparagus
Sweet bell peppers	Mangoes
Cucumbers	Papayas
Cherry tomatoes	Kiwifruits
Snap peas	Aubergine
Potatoes	Grapefruits
Hot peppers	Melons
Kale/collard greens	Cauliflower
	Sweet potatoes

EWG's Shopper's Guide to Pesticides in Produce calculates that USDA tests found a total of 165 different pesticides on thousands of fruit and vegetable samples examined in 2013.

After spending years researching the merits of all the various food wars, food journalist Michael Pollan came up with my all-time-favourite food recommendation: 'Eat food. Not too much. Mostly plants.' As Pollan points out, what all food experts can agree upon is that the standard Western diet is very bad for our health.[6] When Pollan says 'Eat food,' he means eat things that are recognizable as coming from a living source. His tiny book, *Food Rules*, is a wonderful resource of wisdom around food. It includes, 'Don't eat anything your great-grandmother wouldn't recognize as food.'

I also love the practical, 'Shop the peripheries of the supermarket and stay out of the middle,' by which he means buy fruits, vegetables, meat and fish, eggs and dairy, bulk foods, and bread, and avoid all the processed, packaged, artificial rubbish in the middle of the supermarket. Sage advice. And in keeping with the fact that our diet, historically, was low in concentrated sugar, as sugar and sweets were hard to come by, he recommends 'Avoid foods that have some form of sugar (or sweetener) listed among the top three ingredients.' We could sum this up by saying avoid processed foods, highly sweetened foods, and foods with chemicals. Which pretty much eliminates all fast food. And the snack aisle. And soft drinks and sweets. If you're able to mostly avoid those things, congratulations: You've come a long way toward moving from an inflammatory disease–causing diet to an anti-inflammatory, health-giving diet.

What You Should Eat

So, enough about what not to eat. It is perhaps more important to think about what you *should* eat, because nothing will heal you faster and more thoroughly than anti-inflammatory, nutrient-dense food.

Eat the Rainbow

If it is dark red, purple, blue, green, orange, or dark brown (think berries, grapes and red wine, purple cabbage, kale, oranges, sweet potatoes, turmeric, chocolate, coffee, and tea), it's probably good for you. Flavonoids are a group of plant pigments that exert strong antioxidant activity. Flavonoids lend colour and also much of the anti-inflammatory, anti-allergic, antiviral, and anticancer properties to plant foods.

Eat Beans and Lentils

I love getting people hooked on beans and lentils because they are really cheap but nutritionally dense. They're anti-inflammatory, high in protein, high in fibre (which lowers cholesterol and decreases blood sugar), and high in folic acid, B_6, and magnesium. Genetically modified soy has got a bad rap as it is grown widely and added to many 'fake foods' to increase the protein content. The research on the effect of organic soy in its traditional forms – tofu, tempeh, miso, edamame – is almost unanimous in its support for soy consumption reducing cholesterol and many types of cancer. And it's a fabulous, cheap protein source. I always advocate getting much of your protein from healthy vegetarian sources: mostly beans and nuts, but for most

A Delicious, Heart-Healthy Trio

The French have used onions, garlic, and mushrooms as a basis for their cuisine for years. No wonder they live so long. Onions and garlic contain quercetin, a natural antioxidant that also mildly thins the blood, preventing heart disease. Quercetin also improves detoxification and prevents cancer. Mushrooms are abundant in beta glucan polysaccharides, which lower cholesterol and blood sugar. They also stimulate the cellular immune system and are known to prevent and even treat cancer. Not to mention, they're delicious.

people, it is fine to eat some meat, eggs, and dairy. And this is where being bodywise comes in. In my clinical experience, some people feel much better on primarily vegetarian diets. And some people feel much better when they have meat as a more regular part of their diets. You need to pay attention to what makes *your* body hum with pleasure.

Eat Cruciferous Veggies

What, you ask, are cruciferous veggies? Also called brassicas, these include broccoli, cabbage, cauliflower, Brussels sprouts, kale, collard greens, turnips, radishes, and rocket. They all smell a bit sulphurous when cooked (like eggs or farts), which lends to their charm in being excellent sources of the sulphur compounds that assist in detoxification. Their phytochemicals lower the rates of colon, prostate, lung, and breast cancer.

Eat Fermented Foods

Fermented foods provide all of those important healthy intestinal bacteria discussed in Chapter 7. Consider yogurt, kefir, sauerkraut, kimchee (a Korean fermented cabbage), miso, tempeh (traditional fermented soy), sourdough bread, vinegar, kombucha (fermented tea), and brewer's yeast. Brewer's yeast, also known as nutritional yeast, is a condiment nutritional powerhouse. It tastes somewhat cheeselike and comes in yellow flakes that can be sprinkled on eggs, vegetables, salad, and popcorn. It provides high-quality vegetarian protein, the most abundant source of B vitamins in the diet, minerals, selenium, and chromium. It lowers triglycerides and raises HDL, the 'good' cholesterol, helps control blood sugar, and clears acne. The flavour might not be for everyone, but if you like it, enjoy it often.

Eat Healthy Fat

The fat-free craze of the late 20th century was not helpful in that it reduced fats that are actually essential to our health. And fats slow down our digestion and keep us full longer. They are calorie dense, but most people find that they eat less when they have more healthy fat in their diets. Swapping empty carbohydrates (white flour and sugar) for healthy fat is actually a good move for most people.

For everyone, enjoying the healthy fats in olive oil, avocados, nuts and seeds, and fatty fish (like sardines or wild Pacific salmon) is a good idea. These oils are high in omega-3 fatty acids, which are natural anti-inflammatories. Most of us benefit from adding some omega-3s to our diets through foods and, when needed, through supplements. The best-researched supplement source of omega-3s is fish oil, because it provides the long-chain omega-3s, EPA and DHA, that are anti-inflammatory (good for everything from heart disease to arthritis) and do nice things like make our hair shiny and nails strong. Flaxseeds, hemp seeds, and chia seeds are a wonderful source of omega-3s, but they are somewhat less effective than the omega-3s from fish oil. Still, these seeds are very nutritious and are a wonderful addition to any diet. If you particularly want to take advantage of the omega-3 content, keep in mind that these oils are 'volatile' – not that they'll burst into flames, but that with any heat or light, the omega-3s will break down. To take advantage of the omega-3 content, these seeds need to be uncooked, and flaxseeds and hemp seeds need to be freshly ground for best absorption. I usually recommend that my patients grind their flaxseeds or hemp seeds in a coffee or herb grinder and then keep them covered, in the refrigerator, for up to a week. The ground seeds can then be sprinkled on salads, yogurt, or veggies or incorporated into a smoothie, as can intact chia seeds. If you want to use flax or hemp oil, be sure that it is kept refrigerated and in a dark bottle. I like to add it to olive oil in my salad dressings, or it can be drizzled on vegetables.

Olive oil, avocados, nuts, seeds, and fatty fish *reduce* your cholesterol levels as well as inflammation and are wonderful for protecting you against heart disease, which makes them ideal foods to consume daily. It is worth mentioning coconut oil, which is a saturated fat, and therefore solid at room temperature (unless your room temperature is warm!). Coconut oil tastes good and seems to have a neutral effect on cholesterol; it is also full of medium-chain triglycerides (MCTs), which are harder for your body to convert into stored fat and easier for it to burn off than long-chain triglycerides. Those MCTs become monolaurin, which has important antiviral and antifungal properties. Coconut oil seems to improve insulin sensitivity in diabetes and helps with blood sugar control. And it has antioxidant action from phenolic compounds. Finally, MCTs, like those found in coconut oil, are being researched for their beneficial effect in treating Alzheimer's disease.[7, 8] I recommend coconut oil as one of the oils that my patients cook with. And coconut milk, which is full of coconut oil, is wonderful to cook with as well.

To feel good and live long, you will still want to limit unhealthy oils, including hydrogenated oils, my least favourite foodlike substance. Vegetable shortening is an example of these, and they are a part of many biscuits, crackers, microwave popcorn mixes, peanut butters, margarines, and deep-fried foods. Because they contain trans-fatty acids, they may be the most inflammatory and most body-damaging substance in our foods. And excessive corn and soy oils are not as healthy for you, as they provide the more inflammatory omega-6 oils. But some meat, eggs, butter, and dairy fat can be fine for someone with normal or low cholesterol. Get your cholesterol checked if you are older than 40 so that you know if yours is high, either from diet or from genetics. Some people are genetically predisposed to absorb and produce excessive cholesterol, and eating more cholesterol can raise our bad cholesterol levels (LDL). If that is true for you, it's best to limit red meat and dairy fat.

Eat Whole Grains

Refined grains, such as bread and pasta made with white flour, and white rice, are much less nutritious and so quickly digested that they turn directly into sugar. They are the problem foods that give grains a bad name. But whole grains – whole wheat, rye, farro, and spelt, as well as nonwheat whole grains (such as millet, corn, oats, and brown rice) – have a *lot* to offer nutritionally, with high fibre, B vitamins, and minerals. Now, you have to be a

INSTEAD OF EATING	TRY THIS!
Bread made with white flour or added sugar	Wholewheat or rye bread, with any other whole grains: oats, millet, or spelt
White-flour pasta	Whole wheat pasta, quinoa corn pasta, or millet pasta
White-flour tortillas	Wholewheat or corn tortillas
Couscous (made from white flour)	Bulgur, quinoa, or millet
White rice	Brown rice or, even better, farro, quinoa, or millet

bit vigilant because most bread sold as 'whole wheat' simply contains some whole wheat flour, but it also has white flour. Read the label. If it has any 'enriched white flour,' it's not whole wheat. The label should read: 'whole wheat flour' or 'rye flour' as the first ingredient, with other added whole grains (oat, millet, corn, etc.) being fine. And if the bread is sourdough, it means that the sugars have been broken down by microorganisms and it has less carbohydrate than regular bread. And although I enjoy rice, it is probably the least nutritious grain we have available and is very high in carbohydrates. White rice, of course, is the worst, but even brown rice raises blood sugar more than is desirable.

Since I am midwestern and come from deep in popcorn country, I feel compelled to share that popcorn, popped in oil, has levels of antioxidants on a par with fresh fruit and adds an enormous amount of fibre to the diet. Microwave popcorn, unfortunately, has the highest level of trans fats of any food and should be 100 per cent avoided. But it is easy to pop corn on the stove or in a popcorn popper. I particularly like to pop mine in coconut oil, which can withstand higher cooking temperatures without breaking down into trans fats. And, it tastes fabulous.

Also on the list of nutritious pseudograins, because they're actually seeds, are wild rice, quinoa, buckwheat, and amaranth. Because they are seeds, they tend to be high in protein and full of fibre and nutrients.

Eat Fish (Carefully!)

It is clear that eating fish twice a week is beneficial in a variety of ways, preventing heart disease and providing a rich source of omega-3s to the diet. This is particularly the case for salmon, sardines, anchovies, and mackerel – the fatty fish. But this can be problematic for a number of reasons. First of all, we are depleting our worldwide fish stocks at an alarming rate. We don't want to kill off a natural resource as important as our fisheries. Resources such as seafoodwatch.org give wonderful guidance on which fish can be eaten without hurting our fish supply.

In addition, large fish can store toxic amounts of mercury (and other pollutants) in their bodies from eating smaller fish who ate smaller fish who ate plants with naturally occurring mercury. Generally, if the whole fish is no larger than the size of your plate, it will not have a large amount of mercury. The most mercury-laden fish in our markets are tuna fish and swordfish. Keep in mind that depending on where it is caught, not *all* tuna is high in mercury, but most tuna is. A good source to see what fish in your area are low in mercury is nhs.uk/livewell/goodfood/pages/fish-shellfish/.

Third, much of our seafood is being farmed in aquaculture; many farmed fish don't eat a normal diet and are missing many of the important nutrients that make fish healthy for us to eat. And in addition, farmed fish are given antibiotics to prevent disease, which, as discussed, are harmful for us and the environment. Atlantic-farmed salmon spreads disease to native salmon populations and is artificially coloured pink so that it looks like wild salmon – not my ideal of a healthy meal. Not all farmed fish are problematic, and there are some land-based fish farms that are both clean and environmentally aware. Both Greenpeace UK and the Sustainable Seafood Coalition are good sources to check out the quality of farmed fish and shellfish.

Drink Tea, Coffee, and Wine with Your Chocolate

It always gives me pleasure to deliver good news. As mentioned above, if a food has a dark colour, like all of these, it is packed with flavonoids and is an anti-inflammatory and antioxidant. Green tea assists weight loss, prevents all types of cancer, and provides L-theanine, which, as discussed in Chapter 6, reduces anxiety and helps with both sleep and mental clarity. Black tea also has benefits, though slightly fewer than the less-oxidized green tea. Both black and green tea slow cognitive decline and lower C-reactive protein, which reflects systemic inflammation.

Coffee is the number-one source of antioxidants in the US diet – which is a sad statement about the US diet – but coffee does contain many antioxidants. In part because of this, coffee consumption reduces the risk of type 2 diabetes; lowers the risk of stroke, Parkinson's disease, and dementia; and decreases the risk of liver cancer and liver cirrhosis. The downside of coffee is primarily the way people use it. Many of us drink coffee to keep ourselves going when what we really need is a nap, or a better night's sleep on a regular basis. It is also the case that drinking large amounts of coffee, more than five 8-ounce cups a day, can be damaging to the stomach and put you at risk of heartburn, as well as increasing blood pressure and heart rate. For women who are well-rested, drinking one to two cups of coffee on a daily basis is probably fine.

Red wine is also rich in flavonoids but contains a particular antioxidant, resveratrol, that is known to prevent atherosclerosis, or hardening of the arteries, and to prevent cancer. Other sources of alcohol, interestingly, when used in moderation, seem to increase the life span. We are not absolutely sure why this is, but I suspect that the relaxation response caused by a small amount of alcohol has a soothing effect on the adrenal stress response. The amount of alcohol that is beneficial for a woman is one 45ml shot of spirit, a 175ml glass of wine, or a single 340ml beer. Drinking more than this is no longer a boon for your health. And if you suffer from pre-diabetes or diabetes, it is important to know that alcohol immediately turns to sugar in the body and has the effect of eating a piece of chocolate cake. Because of this, regular alcohol use can also cause weight gain from the extra sugar calories. As with most things, moderation is the key here. And just a gentle warning: If you are using alcohol consistently to relax, it is easy for that need to escalate and alcohol use to become habitual. Alcohol is fine when you are happy, with family or friends, and generally healthy. If you are using it to relieve stress or dull emotional pain, it is potentially dangerous. Be careful.

The health benefit of chocolate has been my favourite piece of health news for the last decade. Chocolate is extremely rich in flavonoids and has significant magnesium and arginine, which may be responsible for the fact that eating a small amount of dark chocolate (think one row of a chocolate bar) on a regular basis lowers blood pressure. Chocolate also inhibits platelet aggregation, which means it prevents blood clots or heart attacks. It is rich in plant sterols, which inhibit cholesterol absorption. Most chocolate consumed in bars or as a hot beverage is mixed with sugar and sometimes milk to enhance the flavour. Sugar, of course, is not so good for us. So, the most helpful chocolate is that with the highest percentage of cacao compared to the other ingredients. This would typically be dark chocolate, and the higher the percentage of cacao, the better the health effects. If you want to maximize your chocolate therapy, raw cacao powder, which hasn't been heated and therefore retains all of the power of its healing ingredients, is available at most health food stores. It can be made into Raw Cacao Balls (see this favourite recipe in Appendix A). Be warned, though: The first time I made Raw Cacao Balls, they were so good that I ate several before bedtime and couldn't sleep until 3:00 in the morning. Chocolate, especially concentrated chocolate, has some caffeine in it, and, if you are caffeine sensitive, be careful about eating it at night.

Spice It Up

Many of the spices that we use in cooking have significant healing properties. We have already discussed turmeric, a powerful anti-inflammatory and cancer-preventing spice. Added to the list of spices with beneficial anti-inflammatory effects are paprika, ginger, oregano, rosemary, cinnamon, fennel, cardamom, and cayenne.

Ginger decreases arthritis pain. And in addition to being anti-inflammatory, cinnamon also assists with blood sugar control. Fennel is an ancient aid to digestion, as is cardamom. And cardamom has been shown to protect against colon cancer. This is definitely one of those situations where spicier is better.

How to Keep Life Sweet

Because so many of my patients struggle with the need for weight loss, or with diabetes or prediabetes, I want to give some guidance regarding sweeteners. First of all, part of getting off the sugar train is stopping sugar and learning to love things less sweet – with no additional sweetener. This really does happen if you eat less sugar – promise! But, sometimes, we do want just a little sweet, and what is the best way to do that? First of all, sugarcane itself is not the worst sweetener. High-fructose corn syrup is the worst sweetener for its effect on insulin resistance and its contribution to diabetes. And in my opinion, just as bad as sugar are the artificial sweeteners: saccharin, aspartame, and sucralose. All three of these sweeteners have been the subject of controversial research on their safety, and sucralose reduces healthy intestinal bacteria. However, my main concern is that they are noncaloric and don't raise blood sugar, but our bodies respond to their use by raising insulin levels, just as if we'd eaten sugar. So, as you're drinking your fourth diet cola for the day, consider the fact that you are predisposing yourself to insulin resistance and diabetes, even without consuming sugar.

So what's a girl to do when she wants sweet? Well . . . I would argue that using sugar or honey or maple syrup or molasses in small amounts for most people is fine. If you are specifically dealing with prediabetes or diabetes, agave nectar is a caloric sweetener whose sugar molecules are absorbed just a bit slower than those of the other sweeteners listed. It is an option. And if you need a noncalorific sweetener, stevia is a healthy substitute. Stevia is a rainforest plant (you can grow it in your garden) that is very sweet, but leaves a bitter aftertaste. Stevia actually *improves* insulin

SWEETENERS TO AVOID	HEALTHIER SWEETENERS WITH CALORIES	HEALTHY LOW- OR NONCALORIFIC SWEETENERS
High-fructose corn syrup	Agave nectar	Stevia
Saccharin	Honey	Erythritol
Aspartame	Molasses	Xylitol
Sucralose	Dates	
Acesulfame potassium	Cane sugar	
Neotame		

resistance, reducing your diabetic risk. But that bitter aftertaste can get in the way, so sometimes combining it with another healthy noncalorific or low-calorie sweetener, one of the sugar alcohols, can be helpful. You will probably be most familiar with the sugar alcohols as sweeteners in sugar-free gum or mints (i.e., xylitol or sorbitol). These are the substances that give the sugar-free gums the reputation for reducing cavities – which they do. They range from noncalorific erythritol to mildly calorific sorbitol to just-slightly-less-calorific-than-sugar maltilol. They have a bland, sweet taste. Because they are not digested, they pass through to the colon and can cause diarrhoea. Some people are more susceptible to this than others, so be gentle with your experimentation. Stevia is available in powdered and liquid form at most health food stores. The sugar alcohols are also available in a powdered form, especially erythritol, in health food stores as well.

Food is an essential part of celebrating our culture, our families, and our lives. Food is fun. When we are celebrating with people whom we love, eating is really the pleasure that it should be. And when we choose mostly foods that nourish us, that make our bodies happy, we feel well. And we stay well. I have been amazed that having grown up with Froot Loops and Doritos (and good food, thank you, Mum), I can't believe how much better fresh, organic, well-prepared food tastes. If finances constrict your food choices, start with foods that are cheap and nutritious – cook a pot of beans. Use spices. Grow your own vegetables or make your own yogurt. Simple food is delicious and easy.

I am not a food extremist, and these are just guidelines. I think everyone should enjoy a little dessert once in a while. And it's clear that we all need slightly different balances for our diet to feel best. Remember, listen to and follow your body wisdom, and see where she leads you. *Bon appétit!*

CHAPTER 9

Sleep: Rest and Repletion for Your Body and Mind

I f fatigue is the most common complaint women come into my office with, sleep issues are definitely next in line. And men are no different. Insomnia and sleep deprivation can make us feel (and appear) like crazy people – irritable, short-tempered, forgetful, depressed, even paranoid or psychotic when they are severe. We are in the midst of an epidemic of sleep deprivation in the modern world. Why do many of us struggle to fall asleep and stay asleep? It is often a combination of life factors and physiological factors, and the solution is to learn how to tune lifestyle choices to your body's needs.

Gabriela is a 50-year-old, divorced, well-dressed and very successful high-tech consultant, and the single mother of two teenaged boys. When I saw her for the first time, she complained of insomnia – primarily waking up in the middle of the night and being unable to go back to sleep. I assumed she was too stressed out and that she was probably having menopausal hot flushes that were waking her up at night. But, interestingly, Gabriela was *not* in menopause, and adrenal testing revealed her to be not only normal in her stress levels, but near-perfect. Gabriela actually thrived in her busy, demanding work life and single parenthood.

Gabriela had slept well all of her life. Up until the point that her sleeping problems began, she was a very active woman who enjoyed a variety of sports. However, due to the demands of ageing parents and her heavy work schedule, she had become much less active. She had also started dating a wonderful man – a very good development in her life – who happened to be a wine connoisseur. She had begun having a glass of wine or two every night. Wine is like Xanax – it relaxes you, but then wears off after 3 to 4 hours, often leaving you unpleasantly awake at 2:00 or 3:00 a.m. And when she was sleeping at her new boyfriend's house, she had got into the habit of using her smartphone as her alarm clock – and sneaking in a few emails and texts before bed.

When Gabriela became aware of how her lifestyle choices were causing her insomnia, she began making the changes she needed to restore her natural sleep patterns. She made time to run or go to the gym 3 days a week. She reluctantly reduced her wine consumption, and was amazed at how much better she slept. She now enjoys one glass of wine with dinner, a few days a week. And she kicked the smartphone out of the bedroom. As I like to say, the bed and the bedroom (unless you live in a studio) are reserved for sleep and sex. No work or work objects (computer, phone, etc.). I also recommend keeping electronics, including your television, out of the bedroom. Gabriela did well with her new bodywise prescription and now sleeps soundly most of the time.

The National Sleep Foundation advises that an adult needs 7 to 9 hours of sleep to be fully rested. Teens need more – 8 to 10 hours. Yet, in 2000, the average American slept only 6.5 hours a night! And America is not alone. Sleep deprivation is a problem of epidemic proportions across modern societies.

Unfortunately, many of the characteristics of modern civilization can make sleep difficult. Excessive indoor and outdoor lighting, including looking at technologic screens before bed, reduce our melatonin levels and make sleep more difficult. Sedentary days and excessive caffeine consumption reduce the healing effects of deep sleep.

Part of the challenge of getting enough sleep is that we are working far more than we ever have in history. In the past 20 years, we have added 158 hours to our annual work and commute time. Working mothers with young children have added 241 hours to their work and commute schedules since 1969. And giving up sleep in order to work is seen as dedicated and productive, whereas sleeping more, or at least enough to be rested, is often perceived as lazy or indulgent. Progressive corporations have started to catch on to the fact that well-rested workers are better, more efficient workers and are offering things like nap rooms in the workplace. But most of us are still living in an environment that is unfriendly to sleep.

Becoming bodywise means that when you're tired you, well, sleep. Crazy, I know. Sure, all of us have times in our lives when it really is worth being sleep deprived – like caring for a newborn baby or rushing an important project at work. The key is to make those circumstances the exception, not the rule. Your default setting should involve a strong base level of good sleep, and when you occasionally have to get less than you need, it's important to prioritize paying up your sleep debt as soon as possible.

Getting the Sleep You Need

Getting yourself to bed and making time for sleep are certainly a challenge, but even more challenging is when you *can't* fall asleep or can't *stay* asleep. Here are some of the principles for creating a bodywise, sleep-friendly environment, based on what have been the traditional needs of the human body.

Kick the caffeine habit and limit alcohol. My patients vary tremendously in their caffeine sensitivity, from 'I can't drink any caffeine or I can't sleep' to 'I can have a double espresso before bedtime and sleep like a baby.' Some of the reason for this is that genetically, you can be a slow or fast metabolizer of caffeine, and therefore more or less susceptible to its stimulatory effects. You know who you are. Most of us need to avoid caffeine after around noon to 3:00 p.m. in order to sleep best. Avoiding alcohol, or at least not consuming it for 3 hours before bedtime, can help prevent middle-of-the-night awakening.

Avoid medications that interfere with sleep. Many common medications can interfere with sleep in certain individuals, but won't have that effect in everyone. If you are on one of the medications in the box overleaf, you may want to try taking it in the morning rather than at night. Or, talk to your doctor about switching to another medication, if it is possible. Use your own body intelligence to sense whether a medication may be an issue for you.

Get active during the day. Exercise of any kind improves the ease and quality of your sleep. It can be as simple as taking a walk or it can be a vigorous workout. Exercising in the morning and outside is the most beneficial, as the daylight keeps your biological clock on schedule – awake and active during the day and sleepy at night. Exercising in the evening can be okay for some, but can be stimulating if too close to bedtime. Pay attention to what works for your body. For some of us, a gentle exercise (walking, yoga, tai chi, qigong) before bed can be restful.

Dim the lights and quiet the sounds in your home for the hour or two before bedtime. 'Light pollution' (think big cities with lights after sunset and all the lights blaring in your own home) is just one of the ways that our modern society exacerbates our poor sleep patterns by altering our circadian rhythm – the biological clock that tells us to sleep when it's dark. And in the last few decades, home light pollution just got worse. Smartphones and tablets are often illuminated by light-emitting diodes, or LEDs, that emit more blue light than the traditional incandescent lightbulbs or candles or firelight. And many of us are replacing our lightbulbs with the newer, eco-friendly LED bulbs that also contain more blue-spectrum light. All light exposure at night can confuse your circadian rhythm, changing your biological clock

Medications That May Disrupt Sleep

- Blood pressure medications
  - Beta blockers (such as propranolol, metoprolol, atenolol, nebivolol, nadolol, and others)
  - Alpha blockers (prazosin, doxazosin, terazosin, and others)
- Asthma medications
  - Beta agonists (terbutaline, salbutamol, formoterol, and salmeterol)
  - Theophylline
- Cough and cold remedies and allergy medications (containing pseudoephedrine, phenylephrine, or oxymetazoline nasal spray)
- Antidepressants (citalopram, escitalopram, fluoxetine, fluvoxamine, paroxetine, sertraline, venlafaxine, bupropion)
- Corticosteroids (hydrocortisone, methylprednisolone, prednisone, prednisolone, dexamethasone and triamcinolone)
- ADHD medications (methylphenidate, dexamphetamine, modafinil)
- Thyroid medications (levothyroxine, liothyronine)
- Cardiac anti-arrhythmia drugs (amiodarone)
- Alzheimer's medications (donepezil, galantamine, and rivastigmine)
- Parkinson's medications (levodopa, entacapone, and amantadine)
- Over-the-counter migraine medications with caffeine
- Cancer treatments: herceptin, tamoxifen
- Supplements: SAM-e, ginseng, ephedra, DHEA, adrenal or thyroid glandular supplements, weight-loss supplements with stimulants or caffeine, guarana, yerba mate, St. John's wort, yohimbe, B vitamins taken just before bed

from 'It's night' to 'I'm not sure.' This happens through light's stimulatory effect on the photoreceptors in your eyes – which then signal the pineal gland to produce less melatonin. Melatonin is the hormonal signal of sleep and 'night' in your internal clock. However, light in the intense blue colour spectrum suppresses melatonin to *twice* the degree that yellower, longer-wavelength light does.[1] So the bluer light that we are now often exposed to has twice the negative impact on sleep of previous indoor lighting.

A study published in the *British Medical Journal* reported that the more screen time teens engage in, the longer it takes them to fall asleep at bedtime. Teens with 4 or more hours of screen time per day were 350 per cent more likely to sleep less than 5 hours at night. They also were 49 per cent more likely to need more than 60 minutes to fall asleep.[2] A recent small study of male teens showed that wearing amber glasses at bedtime (which block the blue light spectrum) prevented the melatonin drop experienced by the control group, and improved sleepiness at bedtime.[3]

So what is there to do about this? First of all, avoiding screens entirely for the 2 to 3 hours before bed is ideal. And dimming the lights in your home for the few hours before bedtime. You may want to use different lights for different times of day – lights that are closer to full spectrum for day use and incandescent or other lightbulbs that omit the blue spectrum for nighttime use. And, of course, candles and fires are very sleep-friendly. If you are strongly attached to your computer or TV for nighttime entertainment, seriously consider getting amber glasses or an amber filter that fits onto your computer or iPad. There is a free, handy app that slowly reduces the blue light emitted by your computer and increases the yellow light as you approach evening (justgetflux.com). These changes are important for you, but may be even more important for your children and teens. Disruption of circadian rhythm does not just affect sleep and mood. It also predisposes us to cancer. Healthy light exposure that mimics the light we were born to experience – full-spectrum light during the day, limited amber light in the evening, and full darkness during sleep – can keep us happy, healthy, and rested.

Snack before bed. It is almost never a good idea to eat a large meal close to bedtime. However, having a small snack within a few hours of bed can be helpful for some people. Turkey is rich in the sleep-inducing amino acid tryptophan, which can support sleep. Similarly, casein, the protein in milk, can also be sleep inducing. That warm milk before bed idea really does have a basis in science! A small slice of turkey and cheese on a wholewheat cracker or slice of apple would be a good combo. It is important to avoid simple carbohydrates (think sugar, white flour, white rice) just before bed, as they spike the blood sugar and then drop it while you are asleep – possibly waking you up. However, a healthy complex carbohydrate – like a small piece of fruit or wholegrain bread, can help tryptophan cross the blood-brain barrier, lulling your busy brain into rest and sleep. Other high-tryptophan foods include soy, spirulina, eggs, fish and shellfish, wild game, sesame seeds, and spinach – so there are sleepy foods for everyone.

It is worth mentioning that many of my patients need to get up at night to pee, and this becomes more of an issue as we get older. Hot milk may be a cosy nighttime sleep remedy, but in general, you want to avoid too many liquids close to bedtime so as to reduce the chances of having to pee. Do keep in mind that the majority of my patients who say that they have to get up to pee in the night *actually* are waking up for other reasons, and then deciding that they have to pee. If you sleep soundly through the night, you may find that you really don't need to get up to go!

Take a hot bath or shower before bed. It can be relaxing and also raises your body temperature. As your temperature cools, your body naturally gets sleepy. Most people sleep best in a slightly cool room, so do whatever you need to do to cool your sleep space. The optimal temperature for sleep is between 60° and 68°F. Simple fans for hot weather (or hot flushes) can also serve the dual purpose of creating white noise, which helps some people sleep better. Also, weirdly, while keeping the room cool helps sleep, keeping your feet warm *also* helps sleep. Wearing socks to bed or otherwise being sure that your feet are warm (think warm water bottle) reduces middle-of-the-night awakening.

Love what you sleep on. If your mattress is too uncomfortable, it will interfere with your sleep. You may want to consider replacing your mattress if you wake up in the morning in more pain than before you went to bed. Also, many mattresses release toxic chemicals, particularly when new, so consider a more ecological choice. Commercial mattresses can contain polyurethane foam, formaldehyde, boric acid, antimony (a heavy metal similar to arsenic), and, worst of all, polybrominated diphenyl ethers (also known as flame retardants). These are all potentially cancer causing and can impact the functioning of your immune system. Consider a more natural mattress made from materials such as cotton, wool, or latex. Mattress labels that indicate the mattress is free from toxins are:

- **Global Organic Textile Standard (GOTS):** At least 95 per cent of the mattress materials must be certified organic. Certain substances, including flame retardants and polyurethane (common in memory foam products), are prohibited.
- **Global Organic Latex Standard (GOLS):** Applies to latex mattresses and ensures only organic latex is used.
- **Oeko-Tex Standard 100** (Good but less strict): This label sets limits on the emission of toxic chemicals such as formaldehyde and volatile organic compounds (VOCs). Chemical flame retardants, colourants, and allergenic dyes are prohibited.

Buying a mattress is the perfect opportunity to use your body intelligence. Everyone needs something slightly different in the quality of a mattress, so you can't choose a mattress without actually lying on one. Pick the one that makes your body go 'ahhhhhhhh.'

Try to go to sleep by 10:00 p.m. In the Ayurvedic (Indian) healing tradition, the most restful hours of sleep are those prior to midnight. Remember that our bodies are accustomed to going to bed soon after sundown and waking with the sunrise, so the closer we align ourselves with this ancient body clock, the better rest we get. Now, it is *definitely* true that some people are night owls, with shifted sleep clocks that make them want to go to sleep after midnight and get up between 10:00 a.m. and noon. Ideally, these people are self-employed or work later shifts, as trying to do a normal job that starts at 8:00 a.m. is hell for them. Over the years, I have been able to help some of my night-owl patients slowly shift their bedtime back by 15 minutes weekly until they reach their fall-asleep goal. This can work with regular practice and persistence, but on holidays or gaps in work, night owls typically, well, revert to being night owls. And then have to acclimatize themselves to an earlier schedule again. There is nothing inherently wrong with having a shifted sleep clock, as long as you sleep long enough. It is just inconvenient for many people, especially those who are in relationships with early risers, who are awake as soon as the sun peeks over the horizon. If you are an early riser, it is imperative that you go to sleep on the earlier side, so that you can get enough sleep.

Make your bedroom your sleep sanctuary. It should be dark, quiet, cool, and without electronic devices (especially the TV). This includes your mobile phone, because it continues to transmit signals while you sleep. And pretty much everyone that I know uses his or her phone not just to call friends but to check up on various forms of work. Having your phone near you while you sleep is akin to leaving your work computer open on your bedside table – beckoning you with all of its unanswered texts and emails. It keeps your mind in stress mode – which is *not* compatible with deep rest. And then there is that evil temptation to text and email in the middle of the night when you awake – suppressing your melatonin and prolonging your periods of insomnia. I am particularly concerned about having your mobile phone near your head, as research suggests that there may be an increased rate of brain tumours in people with high levels of handheld mobile phone use.

For some people, electrical devices, lit or unlit, can also disrupt circadian rhythm, as they emit electromagnetic fields. This is not the case for everyone, but if you find yourself sleepless in bed despite all other efforts, consider getting alarm clocks and all other electrical devices away from your bed – ideally at least 3 feet away. If you are not sure whether to be concerned about your electric devices, you can check the intensity of their electrical fields with a gauss meter, which can be found online. Be sure that the electrical field being created by your devices does not exceed the amount recommended by experts.

Earplugs can be very helpful to reduce ambient noise – including snores or sounds from your sleeping partner, human or animal. When our twins were toddlers, and my husband and I shared night shifts, we came to worship earplugs for the deafening effect for the sleeping parent not on duty. Earplugs come in a variety of materials, from simple foam to silicone to custom made, specifically moulded to the shape of your ear canal. Everyone has a different favourite, so I suggest that you explore them on your own. My personal favourite for price and ease of use are the silicone earplugs, though I must admit to sleeping through a fire alarm while wearing them. If you are one of the folks who can't stand to have things in your ears, there are over-the-ear sound-reducing devices available online that work fairly well (check out hibermate.co.uk). And if noise reduction is not possible because you are caring for small children, do your best to reduce distracting noises in your bedroom. Have your partner get support for his or her snoring or consider a white-noise machine.

Kick out the kitty or canine. Unless you are absolutely sure that your pet does not wake you up with its cuddling, moving, or crying at night, you should give your furry friend another place to sleep. You'll be a much better pet owner if you are well-rested. And if your kids are in your bed, they can also disturb your sleep. Everyone needs to make his or her own decision about whether to sleep with babies and toddlers – there is no right answer here – but if your child is severely disturbing your sleep, you will be a much less patient mama in the morning. Sometimes when you are nursing at night, it's actually easier to sleep with your baby. But when they get a little larger, kids can be huge destroyers of nighttime slumber. Do yourself a favour and put your precious one in a safe, comfortable sleeping place of his or her own. The transition can be hell, but the payoff of better sleep in the long run is worth it. And my advice if you and your family are committed to a family bed for the foreseeable future? Get the biggest bed (or platform of combined beds) that you can manage.

Consider essential oils such as lavender or lemon balm. You can use these in your bath, on your skin in a lotion or oil, or dropped onto your pillow for their sleep-inducing quality.

Do not do anything in bed except sleep or make love. If you have no difficulty with insomnia, you can read in bed, as long as it is not related to your work. If you do have insomnia, it is best to read in a chair outside the bedroom and then to go to bed when you are drowsy. Never work, do homework, or pay bills in bed. It is especially damaging to your sleep to answer emails or texts in bed as they (1) wake you up and (2) shine electronically produced blue light into your eyes when you are trying to sleep, reducing your melatonin. If you wake up and can't go back to sleep within 15 minutes, get out of bed and do something relaxing. Train your body that the only thing that happens in bed is sleep – or sex. Especially because sex is a great sleep inducer. Ideally, you should not do work, or anything stressful, for at least an hour before bed. Leaving 2 hours to relax or do simple household tasks or be with loved ones is ideal.

Still Struggling to Sleep?

These recommendations are relevant to all my patients with sleep disorders, but despite these, many women still struggle to sleep well. If the issue is a wakeful mind at bedtime that doesn't want to slow down, there are many possible options for treatment. First of all, exercise and some kind of meditative activity (seated or walking meditation, yoga, tai chi, qigong) can do wonders to train the mind to be calm. The simple belly breathing exercise (see page 21) can be extremely helpful with this. You can also use the body feelings exercise (see page 34) to check in with the parts of your body that are tense or having a hard time letting go into sleep. Can you breathe deeply into each part of your body with the reassurance that you can address all of her fears in the morning? Imagine that as you breathe into your tight neck or busy brain, all of those thoughts and fears are leaving your body with your breath.

Everyone will have difficulty calming her brain in times of great stress, chaos, or grief, but some of my patients are plagued by frenzied and chatty brain all of the time. My go-to treatments in these circumstances are below. Keep in mind that almost *all* sleep herbs and supplements will augment other sedating sleep or anxiety medications or alcohol or prescription narcotics. Please consult your physician if you are on any other medications prior to trying these.

Herbs and Supplements for Sleep

Valerian root: Really the queen of the sleep herbs, valerian has excellent research supporting its effectiveness in getting us to sleep and improving and extending deep sleep and a healthy sleep cycle. Valerian works in a broad range of doses, from 20 milligrams (found in most valerian sleep teas) to 600 milligrams (found in supplements), taken 45 minutes before bed. Most women don't have morning hangover effects, but some do. The other common side effect is enhanced dreaming in some, which could be fine, or not – if the dreams are nightmares. As with all substances, I suggest starting small and increasing as needed. Valerian actually works best if used regularly.

Passionflower: Passionflower, in addition to being beautiful, is an effective, mild treatment for anxiety and insomnia. It has few side effects and can be effective for some when valerian is not. It can be taken as a tea (steep 1 teaspoon for 10 to 15 minutes) or by capsule or tincture. It is also often found in combination with other herbs for sleep.

Magnesium: As mentioned, magnesium is important for energy and muscle relaxation, but it can also be helpful with sleep. A well-done trial in the elderly shows it to be effective for sleep at 500 milligrams before bedtime.[4] Magnesium comes in many forms, some of which are better for softening the stools, if needed (citrate, oxide, chloride), and others that are better absorbed for sleep, fatigue, or muscle spasm (aspartate complexes seem to be particularly good for fatigue, glycinate or l-threonate for anxiety or sleep). It is also possible to use magnesium topically in a magnesium chloride lotion, gel, or oil. Some practitioners recommend applying it to the feet before bed. This is a nice ritual for kids. Taking a bath before bed with Epsom salts (magnesium sulphate) can be relaxing and sleep-inducing.

Other helpful herbs and supplements: As discussed in Chapter 6, L-theanine, Lavela (oral lavender oil), and kava are all supplements that can help with anxiety and with sleep. Many sleep remedies on the market come with a combination of herbs and supplements, which can add to the effectiveness of the remedy. Simple safe herbs such as chamomile, hops, skullcap, and lemon balm are worthy additions to such remedies. Preliminary research shows that California poppyseed extract can be useful for anxiety and insomnia, particularly in a recent study where poppyseed extract was combined with magnesium and hawthorn. California poppyseed extract also has the quality of reducing pain at night, so is a good herb to try if your insomnia is in part due to chronic pain.

When a patient has both depression and insomnia, one of my go-to treatments is 5-HTP (5-hydroxy tryptophan). It is a precursor to serotonin and is also sedating for most women, improving their sleep onset and keeping them asleep. This cannot be taken when you're on a prescription antidepressant, so if you are on other medications, please check with your doctor prior to using.

Melatonin can also be effective and is a very safe sleep supplement, taken in doses from 0.4 milligram to up to 5 milligrams before bed. Because the pineal gland releases melatonin at nighttime as part of setting our internal sleep clock, melatonin is effective in those for whom the sleep clock is altered. For example, studies show melatonin to be effective when taken for 4 days during and after time zone changes due to travel. It can also be effective in shift-workers and in the elderly, who have lower levels of natural melatonin. It is one of the major supplements I use for sleep in teens. It is not as effective for chronic insomnia in adults, but can be very effective in certain individuals and is safe to try.

Could Hormones Be Disrupting Your Sleep?

If you are under prolonged stress, and especially if you are between the ages of 40 and 60, your hormones can *definitely* affect your sleep. And not usually for the better.

Some women have an exaggerated stress response at night, with high cortisol levels before bed, when they are supposed to be low. In the discussion of adrenal fatigue in Chapter 3, I mentioned the natural cortisol curve – higher levels in the morning for energy and lower levels at night for sleep. In my patients who just can't fall asleep, checking adrenal salivary cortisol levels can be helpful. (These can be performed by a holistic or complementary health practitioner.) If cortisol levels are high before bed, in addition to meditative activity, certain supplements can help lower nighttime cortisol levels. My two favourites are phosphatidylserine (that's a mouthful!) and ashwagandha. It must take many letters to subdue cortisol. Phosphatidylserine seems to blunt the rise of cortisol, particularly after physical stress. It also shows some promise in preventing dementia. Ashwagandha is a traditional Ayurvedic, or Indian, adaptogen – meaning that if you need strength and stimulation, it gives you that. And if you are stressed and your cortisol is high, it calms you down. It is a wonderful support for stressed adrenals.

Several changes in our sleep cycles occur as we age. We fall asleep earlier, wake earlier, and are more likely to awaken at the end of sleep cycles in the middle of the night. In other words, we are lighter sleepers as we get older.[5, 6] Complicating these changes are the hormonal shifts of perimenopause and menopause. Beginning at age 40 for most women, there is a natural decline in progesterone levels during the 2 weeks prior to menstruation. This can exacerbate premenstrual syndrome (PMS) and anxiety. It can also disrupt sleep, as natural progesterone has a calming effect on the body. Other signs of low progesterone are warm flushes – at night or during the day – especially in the week before your period, and having unusually heavy menstrual bleeding. If you add significant stress of any kind to this hormonal picture, you further deplete your progesterone and exacerbate all the above symptoms. Stress reduction in any form helps, of course. In many of my perimenopausal patients complaining of these symptoms, I prescribe bioidentical progesterone at 50 to 200 milligrams before bed in the 2 weeks prior to their period. This can have a remarkable effect on sleep, as progesterone breaks down into allopregnanolone, which stimulates the GABA (gamma-aminobutyric acid) receptor. The GABA receptor is calming; other medications that act on the GABA receptor include Valium, Lorazepam, Zolpidem, or the other benzodiazepines. Progesterone is available as a cream as well, but oral progesterone has a better sleep-inducing effect. It is widely available by prescription.

When women truly move into the menopausal transition and start having disturbed sleep because they wake up warm and start tossing their covers off, it is time to address the hot flushes themselves. I like to start with safe, nonhormonal treatments, such as black cohosh at 20 to 300 milligrams twice daily. Black cohosh can work synergistically with valerian root to relieve hot flushes and improve sleep. Isoflavones, such as those in soy or lentils, can also curb hot flushes. The isoflavone genistein can be taken at 50 to 60 milligrams daily and reduces hot flush frequency. These treatments are probably safe and do not seem to contribute to the risk of breast, ovarian, or uterine cancer. If you have a history of any of these, you should consult with your doctor prior to using any supplements for menopause. 2015 NICE guidelines advise that black cohosh and isoflavones may help relieve flushes, but there are many preparations available and they may vary in strength, or interact with other things, so check the dosage carefully. Traditional Chinese medicine, including acupuncture and herbs, can also be helpful with menopausal symptoms and with insomnia, in general.

Progesterone by itself can help with menopausal hot flushes, and I sometimes start my patients with this. When my menopausal patients are suffering from nighttime hot flushes that disturb sleep, and are not responding to other treatments, I use topical oestradiol, in combination with progesterone, if needed, to treat the hot flushes. For a more detailed discussion of the pros and cons of hormone-replacement therapy, see Appendix A. Even small doses of oestradiol can be very effective in preventing hot flushes and guaranteeing a good night's sleep. And when my patients can wean off of oestrogen without severe insomnia, we slowly reduce the dose and discontinue it.

If despite all of these suggested treatments my patients still can't sleep, I consider sleep medications. Generally, I try to limit the medications that my patients need to take, but I can't help anyone to be well if she can't sleep. And, sometimes, when nothing else is effective, a sleep medication is, literally, lifesaving. For example, the first principle of treating patients with chronic fatigue, fibromyalgia, or chronic pain is making sure that they have adequate sleep. Here is a list of medications, with their benefits and drawbacks.

SLEEP MEDICATIONS THAT CAN BE TAKEN ON A REGULAR BASIS

- Trazodone (antidepressant and anti-anxiety medication)
- Amitriptyline and doxepin (tricyclic antidepressants)
- Ramelteon (melatonin agonist) – not widely available in the UK
- Mirtazapine (sedating antidepressant)

Let it be said that all four of these medications have a wide variety of side effects, from morning drowsiness to dry mouth to hangover effect in the morning. They should always be used at the lowest effective dose and under a doctor's supervision.

SLEEP MEDICATIONS THAT SHOULD NOT BE TAKEN ON A REGULAR BASIS

- Diphenhydramine (a sedating antihistamine)
- Safer benzodiazepines (zolpidem, zaleplon, zopiclone)
- Benzodiazepines (lorazepam, diazepam, etc.)
- Belsomra (a unique, new sleep medicine that blocks orexin – a compound that keeps us awake)

Diphenhydramine is the over-the-counter antihistamine in products such as Nytol or Sleep Aid. Until recently, it was my go-to over-the-counter sleep medication. Unfortunately, over the past few years, it has become apparent that regular use of diphenhydramine (and possibly all antihistamines) may be associated with Alzheimer's disease. Not what most of us are looking for. For this reason, I think it's fine to use from time to time, but preferably not on a regular basis. All of the benzodiazepines disturb deep sleep, are addictive, and have a rebound effect when stopped. For this reason, I would only recommend them for occasional use. Belsomra is an exciting new medication that is only available in the US at the moment. It has an entirely different mechanism of action than traditional sleep medications. Because it is new, I would recommend caution with regular use until more data is available on its general reactions.

Medical Sleep Disorders

If, despite all these recommendations, you still can't sleep, you may want to consider seeing a sleep specialist and doing a formal sleep evaluation. Some of the signs that you may be suffering from a medical sleep disorder are below.

- Heavy snoring or cessation of breathing in the middle of the night (sleep apnoea)
- Never feeling rested in the morning, no matter how much sleep you get (multiple sleep disorders)
- Legs moving so much at night that you can't get to sleep or stay asleep (restless legs syndrome)
- Falling asleep spontaneously during the day (exhaustion, narcolepsy, or circadian rhythm disorders)
- Sleeping excessively
- Abnormal behaviours during sleep (like sleepwalking, eating, talking, and night terrors)

Many of the sleep disorders can be effectively treated. If you are concerned about a possible sleep disorder, check out the great information at the National Sleep Foundation (sleepfoundation.org). Treating a sleep disorder can give you a new life. If you need help with your sleep, be sure that you get it.

About 5 years ago, I took a holiday for 3 weeks to a beautiful home in Mexico. I hadn't had such a long break in decades. And I remember in the third week, really getting into that rhythm of listening to my body. I was sleeping when I was tired, and playing or working when I was awake. It was delightful. I had an awareness in my body of what being fully rested really felt like. I committed to sleeping enough on a regular basis that I could be the most patient, playful, creative, and productive woman I could be. And although I am far from perfect, it is now rare that I don't get at least 7½ to 8½ hours of sleep on a regular basis. And weirdly, I am far more creative in my work, more joyful and intense in my play, and sick far less often. Sleep is the resting rhythm that feeds our bodies and souls in the night, so that we can shine our brightest light all day long. I hope that these sleep suggestions help you to be your own bodywise sleeper. You, your family and friends, and the world you work in will all benefit.

Most of the issues that cause poor sleep can be addressed without any medical workup whatsoever. But there are a few evaluations that I would recommend if the sleep prescription above is not sufficient.

Health Workup for Insomnia

- Optimal thyroid function: TSH, free T3, free T4
- Tracking sleep on one of the many devices available for that purpose
- Adrenal testing: salivary cortisol measurements
- If suspicion of sleep apnoea, restless legs syndrome, or other severe medical sleep disorder: a sleep study to be ordered by your doctor

CHAPTER 10

Move: Fitness, Flexibility, and Strengthening Your Body

From our very first heartbeat, movement is the sign of life. What happens when you take humans designed for almost constant movement and sit them in a chair in front of a computer for 9 hours each day and then sit them in front of a steering wheel or TV for the rest of their waking hours? All the common complaints of modern life. Back and neck pain, obesity, high blood pressure, diabetes, depression and anxiety, and insomnia. We were made to move. Many researchers believe that humans, for most of our history, walked 15 miles each day – hunting, gathering, and escaping predators. And it is clear that movement is essential to our well-being. Even moderate exercise, 30 minutes three times weekly, has tremendous health benefits, decreasing the risk of heart disease and stroke, cancer, depression and anxiety, insomnia, chronic pain, and injury.

Like many activities – sleep, sex, healthy eating – exercise has a positive feedback loop. It's easier to want to exercise, once you've benefited from exercising for 1 to 2 weeks. The body learns to crave what makes it feel good, whether it's sleep, sex, or exercise, so giving yourself some of what you know you need makes it easier to *want* more of it next time. This is the positive self-reinforcing cycle of the body, and bodywise women take full advantage of it. For example, when you go for a walk in the sunshine over your lunch hour at work, you get your blood flowing through your muscles in a way that's pleasant and reduces painful tension. You feel happier from the sunshine hitting your retinas and telling your brain that it's a nice day. *And,* when you exercise, your body releases endorphins, natural morphine-like painkillers that create a feeling of euphoria and reduce body pain. Pretty good, eh? And it's easy to imagine that your body's going to want more of that business tomorrow.

So why, then, are many of us so inactive? Certainly the demands of work and home can impinge upon the time available to be active, but it is also true that when we are stressed and tired, going for a run is less appealing. Which is particularly sad, since exercise can reduce both stress and fatigue.

Vonda is a strong-minded patient who came to see me a few years ago, even though she has avoided doctors most of her life. When I saw her at age 55, she had been living in the countryside and growing and eating her own food and using natural remedies to keep herself well. Unfortunately, she was less active than she had been earlier in her life and now weighed 216 pounds at 5 feet 6 inches tall. Laboratory evaluations showed that she had pre-diabetes with a HgA1C (3-month measure of blood sugar) of 6.2, elevated cholesterol with an LDL of 175, and high blood pressure at 140/102. I was concerned about her risks, and we spoke about the importance of exercise, dietary changes, and weight loss. She had some difficulty getting motivated at first, but later that year, her sister had a heart attack, and Vonda became concerned for her own health and much more motivated.

In Vonda's case, I thought it was likely that, with real commitment to diet changes and exercise, she wouldn't need medications for cholesterol and high blood pressure. But to protect her health while she began to limit cholesterol and high-sugar foods and commit to exercise, we started blood pressure and cholesterol-lowering medications, with great results. And Vonda got serious about getting active. At our last visit, she said, 'When I tried to walk in the mornings, I was just dragging my ass to the door, and *so* happy to come home and sit back down. And now, after a month or so, my body is just like a dog – it can't wait to get going. And when I don't walk, I feel bad. It's not a forced labour anymore – it's a love.' Vonda had engaged the positive feedback loop of exercise, and now she's finding a girlfriend to walk with her in the afternoon as well. And adding arm weights. Her prediabetes is reversing itself, without medication. Physical activity is actually *more* effective than medication in reversing prediabetes. And studies demonstrate that the chemicals in the blood that increase with exercise are directly responsible for this positive effect on blood sugar and insulin.[1]

The word 'exercise' has the unfortunate association of a miserable, sweaty person on a treadmill. I prefer 'movement,' as it is clear that simply walking around in your daily life is beneficial, as is gardening and outdoor work. I encourage my patients to get movement into their daily lives as much as possible, so that they don't need to make special time for exercise – as it often just doesn't happen. Biking or walking to work is a great example of this. It's also helpful to do movement activities that you really look forward to – that are fun for you. Many women enjoy dance classes or playing a sport with friends. Or conducting meetings on a walk. Or meeting friends for a hike rather than for a drink. If it's fun for you, and you get that positive feedback loop going, it's a lot more likely that you'll do it more often.

My friend John Robbins wrote a beautiful book, *Healthy at 100,* that describes five groups of people from all over the world that live healthy lives into their nineties, and even more than 100 years. They range from the Abkhazians in the Caucasus Mountains to the Hunza in mountainous Pakistan to the Sardinians off the coast of Italy. In every case, these remarkable people are physically active on a regular basis – hiking, carrying, and farming. Their activities are necessary to their daily living, and they continue to be extremely active throughout their nineties. My own grandparents, who lived on a small farm in southern Illinois, lived healthfully into their nineties, despite consuming large amounts of bacon and pie. I am convinced that it was their constant daily physical activity that kept them strong, flexible, and young.

In thinking about our evolutionarily adapted fitness, it is important to ask, 'What movement are we made for?' Clearly walking, running, swimming, lifting and carrying, rowing, and dancing are movements that humans have been doing for millennia. And although bicycles were later inventions, I would also argue that bicycling involves basic human movement. As do many sports, martial arts, and yoga – which have developed over thousands of years. I do find in my practice that the movements we are adapted for are the easiest forms of physical exercise to integrate into our lives. They are also the least likely to hurt our bodies when we do them with the proper form.

It is also the case that movement while outside is particularly beneficial. A number of studies have found that city-dwellers who do not have access to parks or green areas have a higher incidence of psychological problems than urbanites with access to natural green environments. Not surprisingly, nature has a beneficial effect on mood, and exposure to nature reduces stress hormones in your body. In a recent study at Stanford University, walking through a lush, green area of the campus reduced anxiety and rumination and improved working memory in comparison to walking for the same amount of time near heavy traffic.[2]

Ideal movement, then, involves activity that we were made for, is a regular part of our day, and takes place outside. This would include taking a walk at lunchtime, walking the dog after work, or biking to work or the supermarket. I would also recommend any type of movement that is fun and playful as a natural expression of our human capacity for joy. Dancing, surfing, or playing a game of tennis with friends are all in this category and are wonderful combinations of exercise, play, and community. The body-wise woman, no matter what her shape or size, can take pleasure in moving her body – even if it's all by herself in the living room rocking out to some '70s music (guilty). And you'd be amazed at how much better you feel after dancing – remember, movement is as powerful as Prozac for mood.

Ninety per cent of the benefits of movement happen with the first 10 per cent increase in activity. So, try out the salsa class, walk around the block, or go for a hike with your partner or your girlfriends. Your goal here is not to run a marathon, necessarily, but to have enough activity that you feel vigorous and strong. The amount of exercise we are aiming for is 150 minutes a week of moderate exercise (see below), to preserve our health and fitness. And this can be divided into many small pieces. Some of my patients like to track their steps on their smartphones or wearable technology devices. A goal of 10,000 steps a day is a good one, and this can be achieved at any time during your day.

A note to the woman embarking on a new exercise regime – be careful of overzealous plans! Getting hurt will set back your goals far more quickly than starting slowly. And if your plan is too ambitious, it can be difficult to keep to it. Do less than you think you can, and build gradually, like Vonda did. And although I am a fan of outdoor exercise, having an indoor option that you love is important, too, as the weather is not always conducive to outdoor exercise. Using a gym, taking a class, or following an online dance, step, or yoga routine are all good options.

Getting moving *at all* is the first goal. The second goal is to find a balanced workout that uses aerobic exercise, strength-building, and balance and flexibility.

Aerobic Exercise

The benefits of aerobic exercise, also known as cardio, are *many*. Aerobic simply means a movement that increases your breathing and heart rate, but not so much that you can't sustain it for more than a few minutes. It means 'with oxygen,' and during sustained aerobic exercise, your body is able to increase its oxygen consumption to supply oxygen to the muscle cells. Any exercise done with great intensity (think panting and being unable to talk) becomes *anaerobic* (without oxygen), as your body can't keep up with the demand for oxygen. (See the benefits of aerobic exercise on the next page.)

You can do aerobic exercise gently or vigorously, depending on your fitness level and your goals. We learned how to take our pulse in Chapter 2, and that skill is useful here to guide us as to how hard to exercise. If you are aiming for the minimum of 150 minutes a week of moderate exercise, we can estimate what is moderate for you based on your heart rate. To begin, calculate your maximum heart rate, or refer to the chart on page 172:

Benefits of Aerobic Exercise

- Cardiovascular fitness
  - Reduces the risk of heart disease, stroke, vascular disease, and cancer
  - Improves lipid profile
  - Increases 'good' cholesterol (HDL)
  - Decreases 'bad' cholesterol (LDL and triglycerides)
- Reduces depression and anxiety
- Improves sexual ability and libido
- Reduces insomnia
- Reduces pain response for most illnesses and injuries (including arthritis)
- Improves respiratory conditions (including asthma)
- Assists in weight loss by burning calories and boosting metabolic rate

Maximum Heart Rate = 200–0.67(age)[3]

(This is an updated and more accurate calculation for women than the typical one based on men's aerobic capacity.)

Then calculate what the range of heart rate in the moderate category is for you.

Moderate activity = 50%–69% of Maximum Heart Rate (multiply 0.5 x Max Heart Rate to get the lower level of moderate aerobic activity for you and by 0.69 to get the upper level)

Vigorous activity = 70%–90% of Maximum Heart Rate (multiply 0.7 x Max Heart Rate to get the lower level of vigorous aerobic activity for you and by 0.9 to get the upper level)

For maintenance of fitness, prevention of heart disease and diabetes, and improvement of mood, you will want to do moderate exercise at the heart rates above for 150 minutes weekly. If you want to lose weight, reverse high blood pressure, or improve cholesterol or diabetes, you will need to exercise more. You can do additional moderate exercise, say 45 to 60 minutes 5 days a week (250 minutes weekly), like walking, hiking, water aerobics, or gentle bike riding. Or you can do more vigorous activity in the heart rate range above for 30 minutes 4 times a week, or include the high-intensity interval-training workout described on page 175 for two of your workouts.

AGE RANGE	MAXIMUM HEART RATE	MODERATE ACTIVITY (50%–69% MAX HEART RATE)	VIGOROUS ACTIVITY (70%–90% MAX HEART RATE)
20–29	181–187 (avg 183)	92–127	128–165
30–39	174–180 (avg 177)	89–122	123–159
40–49	167–173 (avg 170)	85–118	119–153
50–59	160–166 (avg 163)	82–113	114–147
60–69	154–159 (avg 156)	78–108	109–140
70–79	147–153 (avg 150)	75–104	105–135

EXAMPLES OF AEROBIC EXERCISE

Aerobics classes

Basketball

Bicycling

Cardio machines at the gym

Cross-country skiing

Dancing

Jogging

Racket sports

Rowing

Skating

Skipping

Soccer

Swimming

Vigorous lawn and garden work

Volleyball

Walking or hiking

Strength-Building

Strength-building happens when you use your muscles to do a task that increases your strength over time. Examples are weight-lifting, squats, sit-ups and push-ups, or rope-climbing. If done repetitively, these activities can be aerobic as well. Strength-building is particularly important as we age;

without it, we progressively lose muscle mass and strength. Having functional strength is more important than looking good, but strength-building, particularly of your muscular core, will definitely help sculpt your body. Building strength will prevent you from getting injured and also allow you to do activities that you didn't think you were capable of. I am a great example of this. I was an athlete when I was young – running and playing volleyball – but had spent most of my adult life as a medical student, resident, and mother of small children, and I was definitely on the maintenance exercise schedule. I felt pretty good about myself if I managed 20 minutes on the exercise bike two or three times a week, while bribing my children with movies. I couldn't run because of foot pain (plantar fasciitis) and hip pain (trochanteric bursitis) and couldn't do any weight-lifting or overhead exercise because of recurrent neck pain (cervical radiculitis). But when a Pilates instructor started working in the clinic, I quickly became an addict. It was the first time I was able to get strong, specifically in my core abdominal muscles, in decades, without injuring myself. And with a little help from a physiotherapist on running form, I started to run a bit here and there. After a year or so, I began playing beach volleyball . . . very . . . slowly, as too much of anything landed me with bursitis or neck pain. And now beach volleyball and running are my main forms of exercise, simply because I took the time to get stronger, slowly and carefully, and avoid injuries. And because I *love* volleyball, and it makes me feel like a teenager, I do it for longer and more often, not noticing how hard I'm working until I sit down afterward.

Even seemingly small amounts of strength-building – shovelling mud in the garden or carrying in the groceries – can have big benefits. Studies show that just 5 to 10 jumps a day can significantly increase bone density.[4, 5] A creative way to build strength and get an aerobic workout at the same time is circuit-training. Typically, this involves a number of 'stations' situated in

Benefits of Strength-Building

- Increases metabolic rate
- Supports independence as we age
- Prevents injury
- Develops core musculature
- Improves bone density

a circle that you rotate through for a particular period of time. Each station has a strength-building activity, such as push-ups, squats, a weight machine, or free weights. Done consecutively, these activities get your heart rate up and are both strength-building and aerobic. Sports that require jumping, throwing, rowing, or hitting, in addition to running or swimming, are also both aerobic and strength-building. Some simple ways to add strength-building to your workouts include doing push-ups, squats, lunges, planks, or star jumps (remember the bone-density benefits of jumping!). Weight workouts can also be extremely effective, but all of these moves require proper form in order to avoid injury. Find a trainer at the gym to get you started, or consider one of these online workout guides to help you with your form and a guide to a simple workout.

- Strength training how-to videos from the Mayo Clinic: mayoclinic.org /healthy-lifestyle/fitness/in-depth/strength-training/art-20046031
- Beginner body weight workout with Nerd Fitness: nerdfitness.com /blog/2009/12/09/beginner-body-weight-workout-burn-fat-build-muscle/

Flexibility and Balance

The third form of activity that is vital to being and staying youthful is flexibility and balance, both of which diminish as we age. Flexibility and balance are essential to prevent injuries and falls. And flexibility and balance will assist in any of your other athletic endeavours. There are many activities that help with this, including yoga, tai chi, qigong, dance, and balance ball training. There are specific classes at many gyms for members over 65 that focus on strength and balance. And some insurance plans even pay for this.

The ideal workout plan includes some activity from each category, for example, combining cycling, weight-lifting, and yoga classes. And, sometimes, an activity has elements of all of these. When I play volleyball, I have repetitive sprints (aerobic), jumping, squatting, hitting (strength-building), and balance training (jumping and turning in the air or reaching for the ball). If you are new to exercise, start with one activity, and add to it as you feel able. Follow your gut instinct to an activity that you feel drawn to. Remember that doing something you love, especially with people you enjoy, is more likely to last long-term.

Ready for more vigorous exercise? A recent study demonstrated that any physical activity is beneficial in extending life, but moderate to vigorous activity (as measured by your heart rate) was even more protective.

People who did not exercise were *six times* more likely to die from heart disease over the 15 years of the study, compared to those who exercised daily or vigorously.[6] That's a pretty impressive statistic! Doing longer workouts, increasing resistance, or pushing yourself harder during workouts will all improve your fitness. This does not mean that more exercise is always better; as with everything, there are limits to what your body wants and needs. Athletes on the far edge of intensive exercise – ultramarathon runners or Ironman triathletes – have some negative health effects from exercise; the intensity can be more than their systems can bear, and they suffer from elevated cortisol and tissue damage from inflammation. I would never recommend exercising vigorously when you're sick, suffering from chronic fatigue, or injured. But, in general, increasing your exercise intensity increases your physical capacity.

One of the hottest areas in exercise these days is high-intensity interval training (HIIT). This is a description of an exercise regime that is condensed, but pushes the body to its maximum capacity for short periods of time, interspersed with less-intense activity or rest. This kind of exercise seems to increase levels of growth hormone (which slows ageing), burn fat, increase aerobic fitness, and preserve and build muscle mass better than longer, less-intense exercise (i.e., walking or jogging). A recent study compared participants who did 30 minutes of steady-state cardio workout three times a week with another group that did 20 minutes of HIIT three times a week. Both groups lost the same amount of weight, but the HIIT group lost 2 per cent of its body fat and gained nearly 2 pounds of muscle. The steady-state cardio group only lost 0.3 per cent of its body fat and lost almost a pound of muscle.[7] It's an exciting possibility for women who want to get an awesome workout in a short period of time.

There are a number of versions of HIIT in the marketplace, and all of them can be completed in a variety of exercise forms, using an exercise bike, elliptical trainer, or rowing machine; running or swimming sprints; or doing floor workouts (like burpees or jump squats), to name a few. Peak Fitness is a term coined by author Joseph Mercola, MD, that describes this HIIT workout: (1) Warm up for 3 minutes, (2) Exercise as hard and fast as you can for 30 seconds (you should feel like you couldn't possibly go on another few seconds), (3) Recover for 90 seconds, and (4) Repeat the high-intensity exercise and recovery seven more times. The point is to be able to aerobically push yourself to the brink of your ability, followed by a period of rest. A good starter workout would be a several-minute warm-up run followed by running as fast as you can for 1 minute, then walking for 2 minutes, then running all-out for 1 minute again – repeating these 3-minute intervals five times, for a total of 15 minutes. Another form of this workout is named after the Japanese researcher on interval training, Izumi Tabata. Tabata has you do exercise at maximal capacity for 20 seconds, then gently for 10 seconds, then maximally again for 20 seconds, repeating this cycle for a total of 4 minutes.

There is only one problem with HIIT. It's hard. Most of us are not used to pushing into our anaerobic threshold (read: panting and feeling like your heart wants to jump out of your chest). This is not a pleasant, let-me-catch-up-on-my-audiobook type of experience. This is why many of the voluntary participants in the studies on HIIT (who are not competitive athletes) drop out. Researchers concerned about the high drop-out rate but looking for the benefits of the HIIT workout developed a slightly kinder approach, called the 30-20-10 workout. Run, ride, or perhaps row on a rowing machine easily for 30 seconds, accelerate to a moderate pace for 20 seconds, then sprint as hard as you can for 10 seconds. Rest for 2 minutes, and then repeat the workout for five times total. Total workout time: 15 minutes. If you're up for it, this is about as efficient as a workout gets. Veteran runners who followed the training for just 7 weeks improved their 5K times by 4 per cent and lowered their blood pressures and LDL cholesterol levels.[8]

Finding your perfect movement. Here are the questions I ask when trying to help one of my patients come up with a movement schedule.

* What do you like to do?
    * You are *far* more likely to continue to do it if it's fun. Love your friends? Invite them on a walk or run. Love music and dance? Take a Zumba class. Have fantasies of becoming Serena Williams? Take a tennis class or sign up for doubles at the local courts.
* What are your current limitations?
    * Remember that injury is the biggest impediment to your activity. If you have a bad shoulder, consider walking or cycling. If you have painful knees, swimming or water aerobics may be a better choice.
* How can activity be part of your everyday life?
    * Can you walk or bike to work? Can you organize a lunch walk with the people you work with? When you are dropping off your kids for lessons or practice, can you walk in that same area? Could you bike to the supermarket or farmers' market?
* What is a doable starting point?
    * Begin with reasonable expectations. You'll feel better if you say, 'I'll walk once a week' and actually do it, rather than have goals that are

challenging to meet in the beginning. Remember that exercise gets easier with time.

* What are your fitness goals?
  ○ If you have specific health issues, you want to design an exercise programme that helps: moderate aerobic exercise for 40 minutes three or four times weekly for diabetes prevention, jumping and weight-training for improving bone density, balance training to prevent falls, etc.

No matter who you are, you can find aerobic, strength, and balance and flexibility training that fits your body, your budget, and your schedule. Movement is the celebration of life. Find your own bodywise expression that feeds your body and soul.

CHAPTER 11

Love: Friendship, Passion, and Nourishing Your Heart

In Western culture, we associate the heart with love in the Valentine's Day sense, but our physical heart has a profound impact on our well-being and connection with others. The heart is wrapped in a complex web of nerves from the autonomic nervous system and seems to have its own intelligence. The heart also radiates an electromagnetic field that energetically affects those in our environment, whether we are conscious of it or not.

HeartMath Institute, a company that uses biofeedback to create calm, concentration, and heart-centredness, has done extensive research on the heart's capacity using a unique biofeedback system that tracks heart rate variability. When we are with a loved one, or even a beloved pet, our heart rate variability synchronizes with them. And being with a loved one takes our heart rates from an erratic, stress-associated pattern, to a coherent one – one that is associated with states of calm and content, or deep meditation.

Not only is the heart 'intelligent,' it may even give us vital information *before* our brain can. One of the most remarkable examples of this is a study conducted at HeartMath Institute to evaluate the heart's ability to have intuition or preknowledge about an upcoming event.[1] Subjects were placed in front of a computer screen that presented 45 random images, one-third of which were emotionally stimulating (violent, sexual, etc.) and the rest of which were calming. Heart rate and ECG (electrocardiogram) and EEG (electroencephalogram) brain waves were monitored, and, fascinatingly, the participants' heart rates slowed *just prior* to viewing a randomly chosen photo that was stimulating. The same response did not occur when the photo was calming. The heart had an intuitive response to information that the eyes and mind did not yet have access to. The brain also has these pre-cognitive abilities, but the heart response is faster, and then signals the brain to prepare the body. This is body wisdom at its finest. And women turn out to be more strongly heart-intuitive than men are. Our hearts literally try to protect and guide us.

Our hearts are vital to our existence, as is our heart connection with others. We humans are a deeply social species. If we weren't, we wouldn't have survived against much larger and stronger predators. We need each other for safety and provision; our bodies are built to crave love and connection. The research on the importance of love, affection, and intimacy is staggering. Whether or not you have an active community of friends has a larger impact on your health than whether or not you smoke cigarettes.[2] As Dean Ornish, MD, points out in his landmark book, *Love and Survival*, loneliness and isolation increase the likelihood of disease and premature death from all causes by 200 to 500 per cent, independent of our behaviour.[3] And all social activity counts here: Friendship, romantic love and sex, a close connection to your pet, and volunteering at the soup kitchen all have tremendous benefits for your health.

The word *love* is really an inadequate representative for all of the vital emotions and relationships that it covers. I can love my cat, my computer, and my mum, all in the same sentence – even though those relationships have completely different levels of complexity and importance in my life. If we were speaking in Greek, we would have at least four different words for love. *Philia* is the warm love between friends. *Storge* is affectionate, empathetic love, like one has for one's family. *Eros*, unsurprisingly, refers to love that involves sexual passion for a lover. And *agape* describes love of a higher order, that is unconditional and requires both commitment and an act of the will. This could be a love for God or the pure, unconditional love that one can have for a child or spouse. There are so many different ways to experience love, each one unique and each one important for our health.

So which types of love are we referring to when we talk about the health benefits of love and connection? Well, all of them, really (except loving your computer – that is not included here). I want to be very clear that *any* of these love types can be beneficial for your health. Have a close group of friends that you spend time with regularly? Awesome. Madly and passionately in love with your lover and having a lot of sex? That works, too. Strongly committed to your church/mosque/temple/synagogue/spiritual community and a regular participant in a prayer group or meditation? Fantastic. All of these scenarios have actual health benefits, and this chapter is about finding affectionate connections with others in your life, in any context. The healthiest people have the most diverse social networks – friends and colleagues at work, mates at the local bowling alley, next door neighbours, kids and grandkids, close girlfriends, and husbands and wives. There is no right way to do this love thing – it's about having love in your life in whatever forms are available to you. It's all good.

A lack of connection with others puts us at risk for a whole host of ills, which you can see in the box below.[4] Our modern society suffers in a variety of ways, but none is as sad to me as the lack of connectedness or affection among people who live near each other, but remain strangers. Researchers believe that we evolved to live in communities of 200 to 1,000 people, with lots of land between neighbouring groups. We are created neurologically and hormonally to know our clanmates – their families and their personalities. Our 'daytime drama' was the drama of people that we actually knew – deaths and births, tragedies and triumphs, and harvests.

Contrast that situation that we evolved for to living in a city of millions, not even knowing the neighbours with whom we share walls. With the prevalence of social media, we can be bombarded daily with the hardships of billions of people, while going through our day without having a single meaningful conversation with anyone in person. To say that our nervous systems are not built for this is an understatement. And our brains and hearts are stimulated, during all our waking hours, by more incoming information from the World Wide Web. Not the comings and goings of a thousand people, but frenetic updates on seven billion. It is no wonder that the young people I see in my practice have unprecedented levels of anxiety and concentration difficulties. Now, more than ever, we need love and connection with others to soothe our hearts, nerves, and immune systems so that we can find peace and thrive.

Lack of Social Connection Increases Health Risks

- Cardiovascular disease
- Recurrent heart attack
- Atherosclerosis
- Autonomic dysregulation
- High blood pressure
- Cancer and delayed cancer recovery
- Slow wound healing
- Increased inflammatory biomarkers
- Impaired immune function
- Depression

A classic story of the impact of connection was the 50-year study of Roseto, Pennsylvania, an Italian-American town in eastern Pennsylvania. During the first 30 years of the study, Roseto had a strikingly low rate of heart attacks compared to the surrounding towns, even though the rates of smoking, diabetes, and poor diets were the same – and they were cared for by the same doctors. The residents of Roseto were descendants of Italian immigrants that lived in three-generation households and were committed to family and religion. Tight-knit community was a way of life. By 1970, the community had become less traditional and less connected and, sadly, the rate of heart attacks rose to that of the neighbouring towns. They had lost the unusual 'heart protection' of their close connections with each other and their community. The heart is not just a pump – it is an intelligent organ with a complex neural net that responds, strongly, to love and connection.

So why do we live longer if we have more social connection? One hypothesis is that social connection reduces the harmful effects of an over-active stress response. We discussed the danger of a prolonged stress response in Chapter 3, in the section on adrenal fatigue. Chronic stress results in prolonged exposure to the potentially harmful hormones adrenaline and cortisol – which impact both heart health and immunity. Studies show that when an animal on its own is exposed to a stressor, plasma cortisol increases by 50 per cent. But plasma cortisol does not increase at all when the animal is exposed to the same stressor while surrounded by familiar companions.[5] The negative stress effect (elevated cortisol) is completely extinguished by the presence of its companions. Its physical connection with its companions protects it from the negative health impact of stress – in the same way snuggling up with your dog or holding the hand of someone you love reduces your stress response when you have a painful or negative experience.

Another study in humans looked at the stress-reducing impact of a strong network of intimate connections – both friends and family. Study subjects with the highest stress levels had *triple* the risk of dying in the next 7 years, but that risk was *erased* if they had a dependable web of intimacy in their lives.[6] Having intimate relationships with friends and family protects us from the damage stress wreaks on our bodies. Being connected to others, emotionally and physically, moderates our stress response – and the damage that stress, and stress hormones, can cause our bodies.

In a beautiful example of how friendship and community moderate risk of illness, a study of breast cancer survivors at Stanford University showed that women who participated in a support group with other breast cancer survivors, during and after their treatment, lived *twice* as long as their counterparts. That is a powerful effect of community on health! These women weren't necessarily physically affectionate, nor were they part of each other's web of intimate relationships. They simply travelled the path of cancer together for several hours once a week, sharing their pain and their triumphs. And this 'support' *halved* their risk of dying. Emotional connection to others and the opportunity to share our pain makes that pain easier to bear, both emotionally and physically. In part because of what I know about the healing power of women's community, I co-founded an organization, Woven, that establishes women's circles in communities across the world (see Appendix B). I want you to have access to many levels of social connection, from touch and affection to intimate relationships to the opportunity to share your pain with women who can hear you and accept you as you are. All of these experiences protect our bodies from the stressful impacts of modern life.

Having a robust social network can even prevent infectious illnesses. In a study of this phenomenon, the Social Network Index was used to assess 12 types of social relationships: spouse, parents, parents-in-law, children, other close family members, close neighbours, friends, workmates, schoolmates, fellow volunteers, members of groups without religious affiliations, and members of religious groups.[7] One point was assigned for each type of relationship (possible score of 12) for which respondents indicated that they speak to someone in that relationship at least every 2 weeks. In the study that used the Social Network Index, almost 300 healthy volunteers were infected with rhinovirus, a virus that causes the common cold, and those with low social network scores of 1 to 3 were *four times* more likely to develop cold symptoms than those with the highest level (6 or more) of social network.[8] Having a broad and active social network protects us from stress, improves our immune response, and reduces all types of illness. We may not absolutely need each other to survive the winter any more, but we still need each other to survive, and especially to thrive.

Take a minute to do the Social Network Index on yourself (in the box on the opposite page). And since we are now in the 21st century – I would include a meaningful text or email exchange (more than 'hey' and not a group text or email) in addition to an actual conversation at least once every 2 weeks in your ranking.

In this study, a low score is 1 to 3, a moderate score is 4 to 5, and a high score is 6 or more. Before you judge yourself or your life (as we women seem to do so easily), I want to point out that it is likely that the quality of the relationships matters – and there is no measure of relationship quality here. For example, we know that women in bad marriages get sick more and die sooner than their single counterparts, whether they speak with their spouse

Social Network Index

I speak or have a meaningful text or email exchange with someone in this type of relationship with me, at least once every 2 weeks.

_____ Spouse/Domestic partner

_____ Parents

_____ Parents-in-law

_____ Children

_____ Other family members

_____ Close neighbours

_____ Friends

_____ Workmates

_____ Schoolmates

_____ Fellow volunteers

_____ Members of any social group

_____ Members of any religious group

_____ **TOTAL**

at least every 2 weeks or not. But having a good marriage greatly improves your health. And having close relationships with multiple family members or a group of friends is probably even more beneficial than having one close relationship in each of these categories. Meaning, if you have tight and chatty relationships with six girlfriends, that is more beneficial than having just one close friend relationship, but we don't measure that effect in this scale. However, even given the limitations of the scale, I have to say that getting a sense of my own web of relationships was interesting for me – noticing where I have easy connections and where I have none. What do you notice about your social connections? Are there areas that you might explore to expand your social net?

You can see why, as a holistic doctor, I sometimes write a prescription for my patients to get a dog. Or to join a knitting circle. Or to go on a girl-friends' weekend. Or to go on a date with their spouse. Or to ask their spouse to give them a massage (it did actually work). It's incredible how much people pay attention to a prescription pad. And here's the thing. If my patient Marion, who is a sharp-witted 83-year-old, actually takes my pres-cription to go to the local nature preserve and train to become a volunteer guide, it will help her more than the lisinopril that I keep refilling for her blood pressure. The friends and community she can develop there will heal her heart more powerfully than her prescription medication. And love and community are available for almost everyone in some form.

In addition to conversation and interaction, some of the therapeutic effect of social connection comes from actual physical affection. When we touch someone we love – a child, a friend, even a pet – the hormone oxy-tocin is released into our bloodstreams and has a number of effects. It increases relaxation and reduces our stress response. Oxytocin also increases the desire for more touch and affection – that positive feedback loop again! Snuggling with your dog makes you want to, well, snuggle with your dog some more. Ditto for the group hug with your friends or the spooning with your lover. Oxytocin also causes the release of endorphins, which alleviates the pain of everything from headaches to arthritis to even migraines. Oxytocin stimulates the release of all the other sex hormones as well (oestrogen, progesterone, and testosterone) – making it a tonic for hormone balance and overall well-being. And we can even get an oxytocin surge from petting our cat or horse, for that matter.

However, I do want to point out that sexual touch produces high levels of oxytocin and all of the sex hormones, as well as the endorphins *and* that sex is a workout to boot – making it not just two for one, but three for one, and a good choice in a choosy bodywise woman's wellness plan. Do keep in mind that sex with oneself does count here. Oxytocin also, interestingly, decreases cognition and impairs memory – explaining why we sometimes have a total lack of insight in early romance – 'He (or she) is *perfect!*' But honestly, a little decreased cognition and memory is not all bad, in terms of your well-being. It's relaxing. No need to fret about the past or future. Okay to just lay back down with your friends on the beach blanket and stare at the clouds some more. A little less intellect and a bit more relaxation is healing for the adrenal stress response.

So how does a bodywise woman get some more love and affection and community in her life? Like Roseto, we can have community the traditional way – large families living in multigenerational households with a close religious community. And that does work. But it's just as effective to create affection and community in your own unique way. Consider your results on the Social Network Index on the previous page. What sources of community, friendship, and affection might you expand or reach out to in your life?

One of my patients, Cassandra, is an artist who divorced her husband 18 years ago, has no kids, and lives alone. Cassandra lives in her home and rents a second dwelling on her property to a girlfriend, who is also an artist. Several other friends live in the neighbourhood, and they walk together at least three times a week and eat together frequently. Cassandra is also a member of a weekend hiking group, where 10 to 20 adults hike 5 to 8 miles in different locations each weekend, and eat together afterward. When I last saw her, she was getting ready to leave for Italy with four of her friends, where she would travel for a few weeks and then rent a villa with six other artist friends from all over the world – and celebrate her 76th birthday. Cassandra is single and lives alone, but she is lacking in neither affection nor community.

Another patient of mine is also divorced, with kids and grandkids several hours away. She lives in her own home and has been dating a man for the last 8 years, who also lives in his own home. They get together for dinner and after-dinner activities about three nights a week. And her kids and grandkids visit her on the weekends. She does work that she enjoys and also happily lives alone, but has both community and affection in her life.

I have friends and colleagues in California who live in modern-day community living called cohousing, where families and individuals have independent living units all on a common property with a shared outdoor common space with community gardens. They also have a shared common kitchen and dining space and have meals together regularly. They host classes and events and have created, through their living structure and mutual cooperation, a small village in the midst of a city. Older and single adults remain connected to the children growing up in the community – strongly expanding the experience of family. This kind of living arrangement may seem unusual in the United States, but it is quite common in other countries to live with extended families in close community housing or in interdependent villages.

You can create an experience like cohousing in your own neighbourhood or apartment building. When I was in medical school, my husband and I lived in a fourplex, and we became friends with the people living in the neighbouring apartments. We shared meals together once a week, popped in for playdates with our kids, and even gave each other a hand with dishes or supported each other during arguments or difficulties, when needed. It was a sweet way to navigate the crazy life of being a young family. I now live in a single-family home, but the block I live on has twice-yearly celebrations and closes off the street to dance and play music together. Not all neighbours are open to connecting, and you may not want to connect with some of yours! But you might also be surprised at how many people are open to the idea.

Beyond finding community where you live, it is possible to reap the benefits of community simply by getting involved in communal activities in the town or city where you live. Anything qualifies here, from bowling and football leagues to knitting circles and group bird-watching to religious services and singing in the community choir. There are a surprising number of organizations and activities available in most towns through clubs, city parks and recreation, educational institutions, and religious organizations. Simple ideas, like setting up a walking group at work over the lunch hour, can reap real benefits in terms of being outside (nature connection), exercise, and social connection.

Being BodyWise in Relationships

So affection, intimate connections, and a robust social network are all health protective. But as you well know, not all relationships are health-giving! Some of them can actually give you a heart attack. Recall the data on depression in women? Higher risk of depression if you're married (especially if it's a bad marriage), and increased risk for every child you have, God bless them. There is no relationship that does not come with some difficulty as well. And we, as women, are generally taxed in terms of our caregiving abilities. So it's important to remember that more is not always more, and that you need to use your body wisdom to forge the connections that will edify, and not overcomplicate, your own life. You may currently have plenty (or too much!) connection and actually need time alone, thank you very much. Or, perhaps you need a different kind of connection – adults rather than toddlers. Or, connection in the realm of play (sports or dancing or just cutting loose) rather than always around work and productivity. Or, perhaps you need more truly unconditional love, like from a pet or a good friend you don't talk to as often as you'd like. And maybe you spend too much of your life nurturing others, and getting a dog would be the *worst* thing you could do for your already-spent energy levels.

I just saw a new patient, Carmel, who has wonderful bodywise intuition about her symptoms. She let me know that several months earlier, she had had abdominal pain and another doctor had ordered an ultrasound of her abdomen. It had confirmed that she had gallstones and this, along with the story of her having pain after eating, led the other physician to diagnose her (probably accurately) with cholecystitis – inflammation in the gallbladder from stones getting stuck on their way out. Treatment for this is typically surgery to remove the gallbladder. But Carmel didn't want to rush to surgery and spent some time reflecting on when her pain occurred – not infrequently after talking with her mother. She had a difficult and abusive relationship with her mother, who was unresponsive to feedback, and calls with her were made out of obligation. Taking a stand for herself, Carmel decided not to talk with her mother for a period of time. By the time I saw Carmel, she hadn't had abdominal pain for several months – the time that she continued to avoid speaking with her mother. Her body was clear that interactions with her mum were hurting her – she couldn't 'digest them' (the gallbladder produces bile to help digest fats). And drawing a boundary with her mum helped to heal her body.

When I met with Carmel last, she was contemplating how and when she might connect with her mum again. It's clear that not communicating with her ageing mother at all doesn't feel completely consistent with her values.

She is struggling with how she might keep her own boundaries around the timing or content of the conversation and be able to emerge whole in her body after the conversation ends. Because her mum was verbally abusive and did not protect Carmel from sexual abuse from her stepfather when she was a child, her mother triggers Carmel, more than anyone else in her life. She is particularly vulnerable and sensitive to her mother's remarks and is trying to find more strength and balance in her current life, so that she is less sensitive to her mum. Carmel, for example, has been a very loving and protective mother with her own children, breaking the cycle of neglect and abuse in the family that she comes from. However, Carmel, like all of us, is in the process of deep adult maturation – how much freedom can she find from her mum's barbs? And despite her dedicated personal work, where is she still vulnerable to her mother and where does she need to set boundaries for her own health and well-being? We all need to ask ourselves these questions in the complicated relationships in our lives – familial and other.

Sometimes this focus on your heart results in sensing pain in existing or missing relationships. The heart connection can also be very painful if someone criticizes you, dislikes you, or wishes you harm. Love, community, and friendship may be fundamental to your well-being. But I've never met a woman who hasn't had painful experiences, sometimes exquisitely painful, in community and in relationships. These experiences make us, understandably, hesitant to jump into relationships and group contexts. Love and relationships are the perfect arena in which to use your bodywise discernment. And if you suspect that being around someone who dislikes you is bad for your health, you are right. Remember those shared energetic fields of the heart? Lovely when they are, in fact, loving. But painful when they are not. The more depressed your friends are, the more likely you are to be depressed. And although extended family units, such as in Roseto, sound wonderful in theory, how many would really choose to live with their parents, grown siblings, and children? There are reasons that some people leave home.

If you are currently in a relationship or friendship that is painful and that you know, intuitively, is bad for your health, you may want to seriously consider altering it or ending it. Or, like Carmel above, take a break from contact for a time. Remember the poison ivy rash Tessa (see Chapter 2) got when she tried to move in with her boyfriend? And Megan's (see Chapter 7) multiple pelvic infections when she was with her destructive boyfriend? What is your body saying to you about the relationships that you are currently choosing?

The benefits of love and community are clear. But in every area of your life, discernment is vital and necessary. Who in your community is not good for your health and well-being? When you listen to the body feelings of your heart, are there people in your environment with whom you need to draw boundaries? You can use the body feelings exercise (see page 34) to help with the discernment of your heart. Often, with family members and with friends, there are issues that need to be aired and discussed in order for the relationship to be constructive rather than destructive. Finding the support, skill, and courage to have those conversations can be vital to your well-being. Often, at least at my house, those conversations need to happen with my life partner, as he has to put up with my losing my rag on a regular basis. We have spent years learning how to be both honest and kind with each other during conflict, and to take responsibility for our own shortcomings. We are *far* from perfect at this! But having those difficult conversations inevitably opens the door to more intimacy with each other.

In our journey as a couple over the last 28 years, Doug and I have benefited tremendously from the strategies of John and Julie Schwartz Gottman of the Gottman Institute, and I cannot recommend their methods more highly, in terms of their effectiveness in having those difficult conversations. A dog-eared copy of their extremely useful 'Aftermath of a Fight' (in other words, what to do when you've both lost it), lives in the top drawer of my dresser for easy access. It is a wonderful guide to understanding conflict and resolution and is available on the Gottman Institute website (gottman.com).

The Gottmans are the foremost researchers on couples in the world, but their methods translate well to friendships and familial relationships as well. As they point out in their research, good and bad relationships are not measured by the amount of conflict present, they are measured by the amount of love, support, and connection in your interactions. We respond to the tiniest shifts of facial expressions or tone when in conversation. Or alternately, we respond to the presence of criticism, contempt, defensiveness, and stonewalling – what they call the 'Four Horsemen of the Apocalypse,' in everyday interactions. In fact, the Gottmans have documented that the degree to which someone is contemptuous, or disrespectful, to his or her partner predicts how many infectious illnesses that partner will have over the next 4 years. The experience of contempt or disrespect from one's partner erodes the capability of the immune system to ward off infection.

You may remember from Chapter 6 that women who are in conflictual marriages live less long than single women or women in positive relationships. Our hearts are connected to those around us for the good and for the bad. Use your bodywise discernment to gauge which particular interactions with those that you care about support or detract from your well-being. The same discernment is necessary with growing children, or with neighbours or coworkers. We cannot choose our families, and we can't control who we live next to or work with, but we do have some control over how often and in what way we interact with problematic people in our lives. Do what you can to process conflict and set boundaries in your relationships. And if you need to put an end to communication for a period of reflection, like Carmel, do so. Allow yourself to find a community or 'chosen' family that supports you to be your best person.

You must draw on the wisdom of your heart to consider what you need now in your life, in terms of love and connection. Take a moment to use the belly breathing and the body feelings exercises from Chapter 2 to get calm within your body and sense your heart. Putting your fingertips over your heart in the middle of your chest can help you focus. Take a deep breath into your heart itself, and feel it soften and open, like a rose, petal by petal. What sensations and feelings arise from your heart when you ask the question, 'How and where do I need more love and connection in my life?' Observe the sensations and feelings without judgement. After a few minutes, use your discernment to try to translate those feelings into more specific needs. Do you need more companionship in the evenings? More friends to do fun things with? More sex? Are you looking for a life partner? Putting intention into who you are looking for and letting your supportive friends and family know (as well as using Internet dating, if you're game) are important steps toward finding a romantic partner. Fully half the marriages in the United States were initiated through Internet dating. And finding more sources of community in which to meet someone also helps. What are your interests, and what groups, clubs, or volunteer activities might you pursue? I've made a brief list of items to consider to find the kind of love and affection you are looking for (see box overleaf). Add your own items, and make your own chart. Contrary to popular belief, love, friendship, and community don't usually just happen spontaneously. They require reflection, openness, and an investment of time. See what kind of love you can manifest for yourself.

Take the time to listen to your heart and pay attention to what your heart is really asking for. When we are bodywise, we begin to tell the difference between the call of loneliness (I need to text my girlfriend for an immediate pedicure party) and the call of the cupcakes. And, yes, people who are in love do tend to lose weight. Funny how that happens, when one's emotional needs are met by people rather than food. After the hideous breakup, it's better to get a massage and a new pet than to have a three-some with Ben & Jerry . . . although I can always get behind a little dark chocolate for these kinds of emergencies. Follow your own bodywise heart wisdom to limit the negative interactions you have with loved ones and to get more of the love you want in your life.

FRIENDSHIP	COMMUNITY AND GROUP EXPERIENCES	PHYSICAL AFFECTION	DATING AND SEX
Coworkers: Go out to coffee or lunch, or go for a walk.	Sports teams or athletic events: local tennis tournaments, volleyball, cycling, or running to raise money for a cause	Schedule a massage, facial, or other bodywork session.	Get *very* specific about the kind of person you are looking for.
Neighbours: Consider inviting them over, having a get-to-know-one-another event with other neighbours, or watching a sports event.	Clubs and associations: environmental groups, local politics, and business associations	Initiate or ask for hugs from friends and family.	Let your friends (and possibly family) know that you're ready to date and the kind of person that you're looking for.
Find people who do activities you are interested in.	Religious and spiritual groups of all kinds: church, meditation groups, yoga, mosque or temple events	Engage in a dance form that is physically intimate: samba, salsa, ecstatic dance, contact improvisation, contra or square dancing, swing or waltz.	Investigate online dating sites in your area and consider getting some advice from a friend or personal coach on how to do this effectively and safely.
Schoolmates: Who are you in touch with, and who do you want to be connected with? Online social networks make this much easier than ever before.	Groups that do something you are interested in: dance, bird-watching, beach cleanup, gaming, 'stitch and bitch,' quilting or knitting, the local film festival or TED talk.	Volunteer to babysit or hang out with nieces, nephews, or children of friends. They will appreciate it!	Consider how you move, talk, and dress. Are you sending the messages you want to be sending to potential partners (or your current partner)? Ask your friends what they think.
Are there family members that you'd like to be in closer touch with?	Take a class: cooking, visual arts, a new language, music, film appreciation.	Get a reliably affectionate pet.	Get active with your own self-pleasuring. Being sexually alive is sexy.
If you're willing, consider hanging out with a mum with small children. They are busy with kids, but generally grateful for adult companionship while parenting.	Homeowners' associations or Neighbourhood Watch	Play a sport where physical contact, hand-slapping, hugs and butt-slapping are the norm.	Take a class that explores relationships, sexuality, or intelligent dating, or engage a personal coach with expertise in dating.

CHAPTER 12

Purpose: Finding Meaning and Making a Living

Having a sense of purpose is the capstone to a life of health and healthy relationships. All of the fundamentals to health are necessary to truly thrive, but purpose offers important answers to the question: Why am I here?

There are some people who have a clear sense of life purpose from a very young age. I knew that I wanted to be a doctor when I was a girl. But even for those of us who know our calling early, our sense of purpose often evolves. Initially, I wanted to be a veterinarian, because as a girl, I actually liked animals more than people and had read the wonderful book series by James Herriot, *All Creatures Great and Small*. I loved the thought of easing the suffering of my beloved cats Ezra, Felix, and Shandy, my dad's bird dogs, and assorted hamsters, turtles, and fish. Then, in junior high school, with the characteristic practicality of a midwestern minister, my father suggested that if I was going to spend all that time and all that money learning to heal, I might consider using it to heal people. I have never lost my love of animals, but I have fallen in love with people and the miraculous journey of helping them to heal. Then, in medical school, I met the mother of holistic medicine, Gladys McGarey, and I realized that I could help my patients to heal their bodies, minds, and souls.

For many of us, our sense of purpose may come outside our work. Even those of us who do have the privilege of doing work we love may find purpose in many other aspects of our lives. There are so many ways to get a sense of purpose and fulfilment: caring for our children or grandchildren, providing income that supports our family, working the soil on a piece of land, engaging in local politics, or creating art and beauty. We can experience the health benefits of a sense of purpose in ways that may not seem grand, but that matter to us, and probably to others. I love this poem of Marge Piercy's that expresses this.

> *The work of the world is common as mud.*
> *Botched, it smears the hands, crumbles to dust.*
> *But the thing worth doing well done*
> *has a shape that satisfies, clean and evident.*
> *Greek amphoras for wine or oil,*
> *Hopi vases that held corn, are put in museums*
> *but you know they were made to be used.*
> *The pitcher cries for water to carry*
> *and a person for work that is real.*[1]

A sense of purpose can be as simple as 'I'm the one who waters the plants outside my apartment building and feeds the cat' or as grand as 'I'm working to end modern-day slavery in my lifetime.' You can feel a sense of purpose from many activities or feel strongly drawn to one. It is also quite normal for your sense of purpose to change and shift throughout your lifetime.

A large meta-analysis from the Mt. Sinai School of Medicine presented at the 2015 American Heart Association Scientific Sessions showed that a high sense of purpose is associated with a 23 per cent reduction in death from all causes, and a 19 per cent reduced risk of heart attack, stroke, or the need for coronary artery bypass surgery or a cardiac stenting procedure. These are impressive statistics and echo the beneficial health impacts of having a strong social network. Now, being a holistic doctor, I obviously want you to move and sleep and eat well. But honestly, having a broad social network and a sense of purpose are equally important for your long-term health.

Usually, our sense of purpose comes from our ability to give to others and to contribute to our families, our communities, and our world. We are deeply social animals, and our greatest joy comes from giving our gifts in the service of others. A sense of purpose gives you a feeling of being necessary and needed – and it turns out that that is very important for your health. We are rewarded, emotionally and physiologically, when we help others. A study of people 55 years and older found a 44 per cent reduction in early death among those who volunteer – more significant than the healthful effects of exercising 4 days a week.[2] And adolescents who volunteer have lower cholesterol and lower rates of obesity.[3]

Having a sense of purpose, like having a strong social network, protects us from the harms of traumatic life events and improves our mental state. Investigators at Howard University studying victims of severe trauma found that a sense of purpose in life was the key predictor of the individual's ability to maintain mental health or to recover from a psychiatric illness.[4] According to a Harvard research survey, those who gave contributions of time or money were 42 per cent more likely to be happy than those who didn't give.[5] Said simply, if we feel a sense of purpose, we are much less likely to become or remain depressed or anxious. A study of helpers – those who help others – noted that half of helpers report a high feeling, termed the 'helper's high.' It found that 43 per cent of 'helpers felt stronger and more energetic, and 22 per cent were calmer and less depressed, with greater feelings of self-worth.'[6]

Why is it that having a sense of purpose and giving to others are so good for us? When we are altruistic, our oxytocin levels go up, we get a surge of feel-good hormones, endorphins, as well as the lovely and addictive neuro-transmitter dopamine, making us want to keep helping people (that positive feedback loop again). Dopamine is the neurotransmitter that increases when we do something that we are addicted to, from heroin to cigarettes to sugar. It is a reward neurotransmitter, and, in this case, it rewards us with feel-good hormones for helping others, and makes us want to do it again. At Emory University, a study revealed that helping others lit up the same part of the brain as receiving rewards or experiencing pleasure.[7]

A sense of purpose seems to be particularly important as you get older. In a study of more than 900 people presented in the *Archives of General Psychiatry*, those with a sense of direction and purpose in life were two and a half times less likely to develop Alzheimer's disease.[8] And in a follow-up study, elderly people with a strong sense of purpose were half as likely to die during the subsequent 3 years of the study. In Japan and China, studies show mood benefits for middle-aged or older adults who are employed and providing for their families or volunteering or assisting family.[9, 10] Not surprisingly, in societies that respect elders, and where elders make active contributions to the well-being of the community, elders live longer and more independently. This is true of Japan; Sardinia, Italy; and the Caucasus Mountains in eastern Europe. In order to live and thrive, we all need a *reason* to live – a sense of purpose.[11]

How Do You Find Your Sense of Purpose?

The markings of purpose arise from the same place as your other body wisdom – from inside, in your intuition and self-exploration. Eckhart Tolle, spiritual teacher and author of *A New Earth: Awakening to Your Life's Purpose*, says, 'Ask not what you want to do. Ask what life wants to do through you.' And this is really the crux of how we find our purpose. Our heart's desire to do something. It almost can't help but do it. It is as if the universe wants it and calls it from us. My friend Peggy Callahan, who has been a journalist, newscaster, and television producer, described her journey to me in this way: 'I wasn't one of those lucky people who seem to be born knowing their purpose. It was more of a lightning strike for me. I read about modern-day slavery in a book and I felt . . . called to help end slavery. Finally. Forever. And it turns out that this purpose is smack dab in the intersection between what I love to do, so much that it doesn't feel like work; something for which I had the talents and skills needed (or could develop them); and what the world needed to happen. Right there. In the middle of the intersection, is where I do my happy dance. On purpose. With joy.'

At this moment in time, I feel a sense of purpose in bringing useful information to you that helps you have the full, vibrant life you deserve through this book. I feel a deep sense of purpose in helping people heal themselves so that they can do their own good, healing work.

Conceptualizing one's purpose may sound a little abstract. So let's break it down into steps that make it easier. The experience of finding purpose begins with listening to your body wisdom. Get a journal or piece of paper and find some time to do these three steps. They can be done at the same time, or each of the three steps at different times, if you wish.

Finding Purpose

Step 1: Contemplate and Brainstorm

What might your purpose be? It may be that what you are doing right now *is* your purpose in the world. Or, you may want to add another activity to your life that expands or carries out your sense of purpose or mission. Or, perhaps it's time for a full life or employment overhaul? Give yourself creative freedom to imagine a variety of possibilities for what you believe your purpose to be at this time. Be open to a broad range of possibilities. Write, draw, or paint your imaginative brainstorm so that you can refer to it during the following exercises.

Step 2: Ask Some Clarifying Questions

Write your answers to at least one of the questions in each of the three categories that follow. It is best not to overthink this. Write quickly, if you can, just letting possibilities flow out of you. No need to edit, nor to show it to anyone else, unless you want to. Mark the three sections on a paper or in your journal, and make your lists.

TALENTS AND QUALITIES

'What are talents or skills that I have?'

'What talents do I want to develop?'

'What talents do others compliment me on the most?'

'What do others call on me to do?'

'What do I feel I'm particularly good at?'

Anything counts here: typing, cooking, cleaning, driving, gardening, organizing people, accounting, building websites, being a loud mouth in your community, making people laugh, helping people feel comfortable – being of use is often not glamorous! And what people need is often not complex.

JOY AND FULFILMENT

'What gives me so much joy that it doesn't feel like work?'

'What do I want to do so much that it feels effortless to get out of my chair and do it?'

'When I lay dying, what will I be thrilled that I did in my lifetime?'

This could be working with a group on a project, spending time with your children, designing and making clothes or household items, selling things at a fundraiser, volunteering at a school or nursing home, making Sunday dinner for your friends, travelling, artistic expression, physical activity like dancing or surfing, raising animals, or building a successful company. What gives you joy?

NEEDS OF THE WORLD

'What does the world, my community, or my family and friends need that overlaps with my talents?'

World and community: Consider things like race, gender, and economic equality, hunger relief, better education, environmental action, community organizing for housing, access to job training, access to better nutrition, better farming methods, clean water, safer bike paths, shelter for the homeless, creating books that educate, building businesses that provide jobs, helping people have better relationships, programmes to reduce violence, a safe place for kids to play, alternatives to gangs, religious and ritual celebration.

Family: Consider making money to secure food, shelter, clothing, and the future, elderly care, childcare, meal preparation, overseeing the education of young people, and being a moral role model.

Step 3: Discern Your Purpose

Now, take a moment to read over your lists and absorb what you have written. Can you think of areas of action where your talents and qualities, the things that give you joy and fulfilment, and the needs of the world overlap with your brainstorm? It's always a good idea to think outside the box. You can reject ideas later. See how creative you can be. You may find ideas for income-earning work, for volunteering, for being active in your family, for throwing your next big party, or for helping your friends.

Here's an example. When I did this exercise, I had many combinations to choose from, but one I saw immediately was that I wanted to do something creative and not at a desk, preferably involving a group of people with dancing and singing. My talents included engaging people and being a good listener. My joy section included deep conversation, caring for my family, cooking (and dancing and singing). And my needs section for my family and community included ritual and religious celebration. It is why I am generally in charge of religious and holiday celebrations in my household – because it's in my sweet spot of purpose and joy.

You can do this exercise many times and come up with as many ideas as you like. As the award-winning poet Mary Oliver asks: 'Tell me, what is it you plan to do with your one wild and precious life?'[12] The possibilities are endless.

I do want to acknowledge that it is often the case that one's income-earning work is not the same as one's purpose in life. I am definitely not getting paid for having Passover at my house. But all kidding aside, a recent global Gallup Poll indicated that about 87 per cent of people dislike their jobs. Which is tragic, given how much time we spend at our jobs. Providing for oneself and one's family financially is a vital contribution, no matter what kind of work you do. Your income-earning work doesn't need to be your purpose in life, though it may be worth asking to what degree you can integrate your purpose into your job!

For example, a friend of mine is a bus driver, and she is very committed to keeping the kids she drives safe and also to being a friend to them as best she can. Driving the bus may get a little tiresome, but the safety of the children is vitally important, and she knows it. She takes pride in her work. And each year, she gets to meet new kids and watch them grow and change. She is a part of the community that watches over them and keeps them safe, which is very meaningful for her.

Another friend of mine is a VP at an enormous corporation in the human resources department. The frequent travel that takes her away from her kids is difficult, and not all aspects of her job are joyful. Her talents, honed in her workplace, include strategic vision and wicked negotiating skills. She has always felt great joy and satisfaction from working toward a world where there is equality of gender and race. Recently, she was instrumental in her corporation's funding of an initiative to match the gender and racial distribution of the United States among its employees within the next 4 years. An ambitious and worthy goal, and completely in alignment with her sense of purpose. This accomplishment, among many others, makes her income-earning work worthwhile, despite its many challenges and long hours.

We all try to find a balance between the dignity of providing for ourselves and our families financially and our sense of purpose and meaning. I remember travelling to Turkey, Israel, and Egypt, and being struck by the fact that no one starts a conversation with the question, 'What do you do?' like they do in the United States. They ask you about your family first – wanting to know who you love. Work is important, of course, to pay the bills, but the focus is on the family, the community, the mosque or synagogue – and only secondarily on income-earning work. In other words, the work of raising and loving a family, or contributing to a community, religious or otherwise, is where most people find their purpose. They don't expect to find it in their income-earning work. As with all things, there is no right way to do this, just the right way for you at this moment of your life. The key is that you find a sense of purpose that inspires you in some area of your living.

Once you have come up with several ideas that seem to fit for you, try out each one of them with the 'Tuning In to Your "Yes" and "No"' exercise on page 9. Do the exercise, feeling your 'yes' and 'no' in your body. Then imagine one of your possibilities for a new sense of purpose. How does your body feel with this information? Is your body saying 'yes' or 'no' or something in between?

A common experience that I have during that exercise is to feel 'yes' sensations about an idea, along with sensations that I am very clear are associated with a little trepidation! That's not a 'no,' just a 'be careful' sign. As we say, fear and excitement live side by side. Some trepidation is understandable with new ideas or changes. And perhaps it would be helpful to build some companionship or extra planning into your idea so that it feels less daunting!

That said, courage may be necessary for the changes that you want to make in your life. And, as my friend and mentor Archbishop Desmond Tutu, winner of the Nobel Peace Prize, says, 'Courage is not the absence of fear. Courage is acting despite fear.' And making changes can be scary. Feeling fearful is not necessarily a reason to turn back. Listen to your body, your heart, and your trustworthy friends, and move forward, if it feels right.

An inspiration on this path to purpose is my friend Lissa Rankin, MD, who discusses finding one's purpose in her book *Anatomy of a Calling*. Dr Rankin is fond of asking, when embarking on a new path, 'If this is what I should be doing, open doors for me. If this is not what I should be doing, stop me.' A 'yes' might look like the appearance of just the person you need to help you arrange for the location for your event, or an unexpected windfall of just the amount of funding that you need to get started. Those who are religious refer to this as an answer to prayer. Others call it a good sign. Regardless, when you are on purpose in your life, there is a sense of unusual support that you get from the universe.

Alternately, you may think that you are supposed to open a coffee shop to create a centre for community building, but the location falls through at the last minute and the bank won't give you funding, and when working on the business, you get a horrible flu. You may discern this as a 'no' from the universe – and you'll have to decide what the 'no' is to. The particular idea, the current plan, the timing, whatever. This is not to say that you should give up at the first obstacle. Often, what is worth doing requires going through times of enormous adversity. Again, pay attention to your body. You are the tuning fork to the universe. Do the obstacles energize you and fill you with greater commitment? Or do you feel defeated and drained?

If doors keep closing on your idea, it is worth paying attention. My friend, social activist Nikki Sylvestri, likes to say that when she continues in a path that is not 'on purpose' for her, she gets a 'bitch slap' from the universe. I know you know what I'm talking about. It's like Tessa in Chapter 2, who got poison ivy all over her arms while attempting to move her clothes into her boyfriend's apartment. Her body was screaming, 'Don't do it! Wrong guy!' When you listen, your body talks. And when you really listen, the universe talks, too. When I met my husband, I had a dream that he was safe for me, and I took his hand and felt incredible joy. And then, on the night of our first date, every single one of my six roommates was weirdly away from our college house that night (which never happened again), so we had privacy and could talk late into the night. My body intelligence and the universe conspired to put us together. And we're still happily together.

For years, I have thought of the 'Why are we here?' of life as a tripartite concept: one-third to learn and grow, one-third to serve and help others, and one-third to celebrate and enjoy. Ideally, your purpose allows you to do all of these things. I do believe that playfulness and a sense of joy are vital to giving life to and sustaining our serving and growing. Being bodywise in our choices allows us to sustain our giving and service in a way that keeps us from giving beyond our means, and overdrawing the bank account of our wellness. A real purpose leaves room for connectedness with others, love and laughter, movement, sleep, and good food within the giving and serving. We want our good work in the world to be sustainable, so we must sustain ourselves. Or, we're going to get a 'bitch slap from the universe.' And contrary to the stereotype of the hero's journey, you do not have to fulfil your purpose alone! Find your tribe, and keep your loved ones near as you do your work in the world. Listen to the language of your body and watch closely the universe around you. Let your purpose unfold from your well-tended body, mind, and soul.

Our BodyWise World

Thank you so much for joining me on this sacred journey to find the body wisdom that resides within each one of us. It has been a pleasure, a deep learning, and a healing journey for me to have had the privilege of writing this book. I hope that the book is an inspiration and companion for you as you live into the life that you deserve. I hope you will return to this book when you need it as a healing companion and a resource for your health and well-being. Health is never static. It is a dynamic, unfolding process, and your health needs will change over the course of your life.

I developed the 28-Day Plan that follows (with the help of my patients) so that you have a guideline for putting the changes discussed in *BodyWise* into practice in your own life. It is a guideline – not a fixed plan – because it requires that you use your body intelligence at every point in the plan to choose the action that your body uniquely needs to heal and become whole.

I hope by now that you are on your way to having a life guided by your own body wisdom. In this book I have tried to help you to:

- Listen to your body wisdom as your first resource and respect it. Your sensations, your feelings, and the discernment of your own mind and soul. This is a minute-by-minute process, and can liberate you to walk your path with gratitude, love, and joy.
- Understand that your symptoms are the key information that unlocks your transformation from chronic body depletion into vitality, repletion, and wholeness.
- Use your discernment to choose people, practitioners, and treatments that can support you to feel healthy and whole.

- Eat living, nutrient-rich food that gives your body what she needs to thrive.
- Find deep sleep and restoration.
- Let your body move, play, and find pleasure, so that she is flexible, strong and resilient.
- Embrace intimate friends and communities that support you to be your best self.
- Live into your purpose and your particular gifts here on earth – we need you.

These messages are fundamental to healing ourselves, but they have a greater legacy as well. They are actually fundamental to healing our families, our communities, and our world. I feel it is my purpose to help you and all women heal what ails them and find their joy, love, and contribution in the world. In my years of caring for women at the turning points of their lives, I've noticed that when they are listening carefully to what their body needs, some remarkable things happen. In creative, individual ways, women use their full body intelligence and capacity to weave amazing work in their communities and in the world at large. When we women recover ourselves from chronic body depletion and power ourselves with the five fundamentals of health, we are capable of beautiful feats of healing and reparation in our world.

We are at a pivotal moment in the history of our planet and our human communities. There are signs of optimism – cooperation, creativity, communication, and human potential – that are new and inspiring. The Internet, the mobile phone network, and a generation of connected young people have created the largest opportunity for global participation and cooperation that the world has ever seen. And I continue to be awed and inspired by the visionary and creatively powered generation coming of age today. They are more tolerant, more diverse, and more solidly grounded in community and friendship than any previous generation to date. Women have access to government, leadership, and education at an unprecedented level. And the innovative potential for crowdsourcing solutions to the world's problems in our interconnected world is exciting and inspiring.

At the same time, we have serious global issues that challenge our very existence. Life expectancy has begun to decline in most developed nations due to the excesses of our culture. The destruction of native forests, native peoples, native habitats, and native wisdom is a real threat to our ability to survive on the planet. Climate change is a threat to all peoples, especially the most vulnerable, and to the animal and plant worlds as well. Fresh water is about to become a scarce resource. The economic divide between rich and poor continues to grow, with hunger and homelessness more common, and our democracies destabilized by these unfair disparities. Despite the outlawing of slavery worldwide, these economic conditions have resulted in the enslavement of the largest number of people in the history of the planet. And as a part of our greed and desperation, we continue to extinguish plant and animal species whose diverse contributions to our ability to survive we don't yet fully grasp. War and terrorism have created enormous refugee communities and a generation of children raised in instability and fear. And women remain second-class citizens, without education, rights of ownership, religious freedom, or even sovereignty over their own bodies, in many places in the world.

I believe that women, with our great capacity for compassion and our connection to our bodies and to the earth itself, will be responsible for leading the next stage of global change. We are needed. Every single one of us, in each of our individual lives and spheres of influence, is necessary to transform our world. And this transformation won't happen because single, isolated women of influence will bring it about – it will happen because all of us, we as a global community of women, will embrace our strength and intelligence and make a stand for what really matters. For our shared humanity. That everyone, each child born on this spinning planet, has a right to eat, sleep, move, love, and find his or her purpose in the world. That each one of us is a necessary part of this burgeoning human family of 7 billion. That all of us deserve a chance to be healthy and whole.

You deserve to have a life of health, love, passion, and purpose. To be bodywise and whole. And when you heal yourself, you heal a vital piece of our broken world. When you embrace the truly unique and amazing being that you are, you allow all of those around you to do the same. And when you connect to the deep body wisdom within you, you connect to the essence of the earth itself. When you choose healthy foods to eat, such as produce that is local and organic, you heal the land you live on, and the bees that pollinate the food, and the animals that eat the insects, and so on . . . . Whenever we make bodywise choices for our own health, we make wise choices for the earth as well.

The native elders of every tribe on this planet know, deep in their bones, that we humans are intimately connected to the earth. That we are part of the earth herself. And that when we heal ourselves and our communities, we heal the earth. We cannot separate the 'microbiome,' or healthy bacteria in your gut, and the 'microbiome' of the soil – they are entwined. We cannot separate your healthy respiratory system and the cleanliness of the air you breathe. Your sound sleep and the light pollution outside your bedroom window. The chemicals poisoning your garden or the neighbouring field and the resulting increase in your body's risk of cancer.

We, and the planet, are both fragile and resilient. When you step into your particular place on this earth, and live a life that your body loves, and express your unique purpose, you build a bond that creates the possibility of healing for all of us.

Thank you for joining me on this bodywise journey.

Blessings on your own unique and magnificent healing journey.

Blessings on our journey together.

BodyWise 28-Day Plan

The BodyWise 28-Day Plan is designed to help you put into practice the principles of being bodywise. It is anchored in the most advanced health science and the belief that you can develop a sense of what your body needs on a day-to-day basis. Each week will focus on one of the fundamentals of health – eat, sleep, move, and love and purpose – tuning in closely to your body wisdom and gently adjusting behaviours as we go.

You will also use your scores on the quizzes that you took in Chapters 3 to 7, so let's gather that data here.

Chapter 3   Fatigue Quiz: _____

Chapter 4   Chronic Pain Quiz: _____

Chapter 5   Libido Quiz: _____

Chapter 6   Depression Quiz: _____

               Anxiety Quiz: _____

Chapter 7   Allergies and Autoimmune Quiz: _____

Getting Ready

You will be eliminating some foods that you may be used to eating, and possibly caffeine and alcohol as well, so choosing a favourable time to do the 28-day plan is important. Removing toxic, inflammatory, or even allergenic foods from your diet can make an enormous difference to how well you feel. Think of eating as taking medicine, with each ingredient in your food sending its own signal to the body's physiology. Just one fast-food meal tells your body to increase inflammation, pain, cholesterol levels, blood pressure, and possibly depression. You want to give your body the eating foundation it needs to signal health, vitality, and happiness. Prepping your kitchen can be helpful! Take a look at the first week's recommendations so that you have time to get rid of the items you don't want around during your BodyWise 28-Day Plan. You may want to stock up on the foods you'll be eating if you don't already have them, along with any supplements you want to include. If you need guidance or inspiration, check out 'BodyWise Shopping List,' starting on page 210. Choose whatever items appeal to you. Also, check out the section on caffeine and alcohol so that you can plan for your intake and wean yourself down from your current caffeine intake, if you need to.

Daily Practice

Each morning of your 28-day plan, take a few minutes to do a bodywise check-in. You can sit in a comfortable chair or simply lie in bed when you wake and do a body scan. The exercises in Chapter 2 can be wonderful touchstones for this practice.

Exercise 3: Body Awareness (page 30)

Exercise 4: Quality of Sensation (page 32)

Exercise 5: Body Feelings (page 34)

What parts of your body need your attention today? Are you waking up energized or especially exhausted? Do you feel anxious and stressed? How can you start each day with an intention to care for yourself in the rush of your life?

During the 1st week, you will explore a healthy eating plan that matches your body's needs and speeds you toward healing and vitality. In the 2nd week, you'll continue your eating plan and also focus on getting enough refreshing sleep. In the 3rd week, you'll customize your movement or exercise plan. You'll continue with your eating, sleeping, and exercise plan as you move into your 4th week, where you'll focus on having the kind of love, community, and purpose that you deserve.

The biggest barrier for my patients while doing the 28-day plan was their expectation that they should do it *perfectly*. That they should follow the plan exactly and never stray from its guidelines, regardless of whatever else was happening in their lives. The most central and most important part of this plan is that you listen to *your* body intelligence while doing it. Which means that if I suggest that you eat nuts and avocados, but you feel lousy when you eat nuts and avocados, you don't eat them! And if you've planned a rigorous exercise programme but are suddenly ill with a cold, you rest instead. The primary guide in your 28-day plan is *your* body.

The second biggest barrier for my patients is feeling that they have to do it comprehensively or not at all. My experience is that all of the aspects of the 28-day plan are important, but each one individually has important gifts to give, and you can choose to do just one or two of the week-long sections. Or you can extend the plan and do it at a slower pace if you'd like. You can also decide that now is not the time to do one of the sections, and simply focus on the others. In other words, there is no *right* way to do the 28-day plan, just the way that works best for you at this time.

And finally, despite all of the best intentions, we all fail to meet our own expectations from time to time. Perhaps you really wanted to give up sugar, but forgot while distracted at work and reached into the sweetie bowl. A sense of ease and self-forgiveness is essential in this process. 'Whoops! I didn't mean to do that. I'm going to try not to eat sugar for the rest of today.' Each of us is learning to listen closely to our own body intelligence, and it is a work in progress. And being patient and loving

Basic BodyWise Eating Plan

* As much as possible, eat foods grown or raised without pesticides, hormones, or antibiotics.
  * Avoid nonorganic dairy and meat (as they concentrate pesticides, hormones, and antibiotics).
  * Eat organic produce whenever possible, avoiding the nonorganic produce with the highest pesticide content (see table on page 143).
* Eat 5 to 10 servings of fruits and vegetables daily, with an emphasis on green, red, and orange vegetables. You cannot eat too many green vegetables! Go crazy with the leafy greens. A serving of vegetables is 120ml cooked vegetables or 1 cup raw vegetables or chopped fruit. A serving of fruit is one medium apple, pear, or orange, or 15 grapes.
* Eat protein with every meal.
  * For one or two meals a day, eat a vegetable protein: beans, legumes, nuts, or seeds. Think nut butter on wholegrain bread, hummus with veggies or crackers, lentil soup, or soy protein like tofu, tempeh, or edamame. (Be sure the soy is organic and non-GMO, not a genetically modified version of soy.)
  * Eat cold-water fish (that is sustainable and low in mercury) and some organic lean meat, with a preference for chicken and turkey. Enjoy organic, grass-fed beef or bison, or organic pork once or twice a week.
  * Organic eggs can be eaten daily if your cholesterol is good, or limited to two egg yolks weekly, if your cholesterol is high.
  * If your body likes dairy products, eat organic. Eating yogurt and kefir helps with healthy probiotics. Some hard cheeses, such as Parmesan,

with yourself in the process of developing your body intelligence is paramount.

Week 1

This week, you are going to focus on eating. As always, I want you to be bodywise in your choices for your own personalized wellness plan. I will make general recommendations, but if you *know* that you are sensitive to a food, I recommend, by all means, don't eat it! Your body gets the final say here! I've included the 'Basic BodyWise Eating Plan' (below) for you to use as a guide to how you eat during this 28-day programme. I would strongly suggest that you consider clearing out the foods noted in 'Foods to Avoid and Limit' (see page 209) from your cupboards and refrigerator, if at all

Romano, or goat's cheese (higher in protein and lower in lactose), can be a lovely part of a healthy diet. Excessive cheese, cream, or butter is not generally good for you, as they are high in cholesterol and can be inflammatory.

- Eat good fats like olives and olive oil, nuts and seeds, and avocados. Enjoy coconut as a cooking oil or coconut milk in foods in moderation. These are healthy fats but are, of course, high in calories. *Do* eat them, but if you are trying to lose weight, watch your quantity!

- Eat organic whole grains, if your body likes them. Think truly whole wheat or rye bread or crackers (check the label for wheat flour that is not 'whole wheat' as it is often there!). Sourdough bread is an even healthier choice, as it lowers the sugar content. You can also eat bulgur, oats and oatmeal, barley, millet, organic cornbread and tortillas, and brown rice. You may also want to try the 'nongrains' quinoa, amaranth, and buckwheat. I would recommend limiting grains to one to two servings daily. And, if you want to limit gluten, see the list of gluten-free grains in the shopping list.

- Limit natural sweets or sweeteners, including small amounts of honey, maple syrup, agave nectar, or dates. Avoid refined cane sugar.

- Drink mostly water. You can add to this any vegetable juice that you enjoy, but limit fruit juices, as they are high in sugar. Herbal teas are wonderful as well. And, if you are not prediabetic or diabetic, a slightly sweetened probiotic drink, such as kefir, kombucha, or jun can be delicious and healthy. Note: Not everyone likes these – it's a particular taste! Be aware if you are avoiding caffeine that kombucha may have caffeinated tea in it.

possible, prior to starting the programme. If you have a family member or roommate who opposes this, you can put those foods in a special, sealed-off place – in a bag or box or cabinet that you don't see. The sight of tempting unhealthy food is difficult when you're trying to eat well!

Do take a trip to the supermarket with these guidelines in mind so that you can start off with a variety of delicious things to eat that are also good for you. It is almost always useful to make a list, especially if you are making changes in your eating habits. Use the sample, comprehensive shopping list as a guideline to choose from. Also keep in mind that you are focusing on fresh foods, and these are typically found around the perimeter of the supermarket. The only thing you would want to buy frozen are vegetables and fruits. Avoid the packaged foods in the middle of the store. And get used to reading the labels on anything in a package or can.

It is true that buying healthier, organic food is often more expensive. I would argue that if you can afford it, it is worth it for your long-term health. And I am also an expert on limiting cost, having fed a hungry family of five this way for decades. Beans and soups cooked at home are cheap and filling. Substituting vegetable proteins (beans and nuts) for expensive organic meats also helps cut costs. You can often negotiate deals with local farmers at farmers' markets for 'bruised' or imperfect organic fruits and vegetables. I have many friends who buy one-quarter of a grass-fed cow to put in the deep freezer and use all winter. You can get fish at the wholesaler fresh out of the ocean, and there are community-supported fisheries that will ship sustainable fish to your home. Using an online company, like Abel & Cole, that allows you to have fresh, seasonal organic produce delivered to you on a weekly basis for a discount. And if you're lucky enough to have some outdoor space, you can grow a wide variety of greens, veggies, and fruits, depending on your climate. Having a garden was the only way I could afford to feed my twin girls organic tomatoes when they were growing up, but it was worth it; I sent them out into the fenced-in garden to graze on the cherry tomatoes, which they still eat like sweets.

Check out the 'Basic BodyWise Eating Plan' on the previous two pages. Then, read the possible 'add-ons' to your dietary plan, depending on your bodywise intuition and your health as assessed in the quizzes. It is ideal to have some kind of protein with every meal and snack to sustain your energy levels and even out blood sugar. Beans, nuts, cheese, or healthy meat are all fine. Most of us need at least three meals a day, and the most important meal for energy (and for weight loss) is breakfast. It doesn't need to be fancy (a little yogurt, a smoothie, peanut butter toast), but try to eat something every morning. This is not necessarily a weight-loss diet, but if you are try-

Foods to Avoid and Limit

AVOID

- All fast-food restaurant foods
- Deep-fried foods
- Soft drinks and sweets (with the exception of a few ounces of dark chocolate)
- Hydrogenated or partially hydrogenated oils (often in margarine, crackers, crisps, packaged baked goods, and bagged and boxed snacks)
- High-fructose corn syrup (in many soft drinks and packaged desserts)
- Artificial sweeteners (saccharin, aspartame, and sucralose)
- Processed foods, including commercially prepared and packaged foods with artificial flavours, colouring, preservatives, and salt and sugar. Think: frozen dinners and snacks, most 'convenience foods,' and foods that have ingredients that you don't recognize.

LIMIT

- Cane sugar (also listed as sucrose, glucose, maltose, dextrose, lactose, fructose) and concentrated sweeteners (brown rice syrup, honey, maple syrup, molasses). No more than 1 to 2 teaspoons daily, and avoid if you want to lose weight or if you have prediabetes or diabetes.
- White potatoes, white rice, white flour no more than once a week, and avoid if you want to lose weight or have prediabetes or diabetes. You may want to consider using the natural sugar-free sweeteners discussed in Chapter 8.

ing to lose weight, concentrating most of your calories into breakfast and lunch and avoiding eating a large meal before bed can help. And many of us do better eating every 2 to 3 hours, so if you know you're a grazer, in addition to your three meals, have some healthy snacks mid-morning and mid-afternoon. For example, a handful of nuts and an apple, or carrots and hummus, or crackers and cheese.

You can be successful at bodywise eating by following your own body intelligence about when, what, and how much to eat. Ideally, this is how we all learn to care for ourselves best. And, it is also true that some of us have a slower metabolism than others and have to be more careful about portion sizes. If you are one of the women who look at a doughnut and gain a pound, you will want to be careful about the amount of grains, sweeteners, and fats you consume.

BodyWise Shopping List

Fresh Vegetables

Green Veggies (mostly)

- Broccoli
- Artichokes
- Asian greens
- Asparagus
- Brussels sprouts
- Cabbage
- Cauliflower
- Celery

- Collard greens
- Cucumbers
- Green beans
- Leafy greens
  chard
  kale
  mustard greens
- Lettuce

- Okra
- Peas
- Spinach
- Sugar snap peas
- Snow peas
- Courgettes and summer squash

Orange and Red Veggies

- Beetroot
- Carrots
- Kombucha
- Red cabbage

- Rhubarb
- Sweet potatoes and yams

- Winter squash
  acorn
  butternut
  pumpkin

Brown and White Veggies

- Jicama
- Kohlrabi

- Mushrooms
- Parsnips

- Radishes and other roots
- Turnips

Nightshade Veggies (can be troublesome with arthritis)

- Aubergines
- Paprika
- Peppers (both sweet and spicy)

- Tomatoes (actually a fruit!)
- Tomatillos

- Goji berries (also a fruit)
- White potatoes (limit number due to high sugar effect)

Veggies for Flavouring

- Garlic
- Ginger root
- Fennel

- Fresh herbs
  basil
  coriander
  mint
  oregano

  parsley
  rosemary
  thyme
- Leeks
- Onions

Vegetable Starches (to be eaten in moderation)

- Corn

- Plantain (actually a fruit!)

- Taro
- White potatoes

Dairy or Dairy Substitutes

- Cottage cheese
- Kefir
- Yogurt
- Organic milk
- Organic cheeses (to be eaten in moderation)
- Organic half-and-half (if your cholesterol is good)

Dairy-Free Products

- Non-dairy cheeses (soy, rice, almond)
- Non-dairy milks (almond, coconut, soy, oat, hemp, rice, hazelnut, cashew)
- Non-dairy yogurts (almond, coconut, soy)

Fresh Fruit

- Apples
- Apricots
- Asian pears
- Berries
  - *acai*
  - *blackberries*
  - *blueberries*
  - *goji*
  - *olallieberries*
  - *raspberries*
  - *strawberries*
- Cherries
- Citrus
  - *grapefruit*
  - *lemons*
  - *oranges*
  - *pomelos*
  - *tangerines*
- Figs
- Grapes
- Kiwifruit
- Melons
  - *canary*
  - *cantaloupe*
  - *galia*
  - *honeydew*
  - *watermelon*
- Nectarines
- Peaches
- Pears
- Persimmons
- Plums
- Pomegranates

Tropical Fruits

- Bananas
- Guava
- Mangoes
- Papayas
- Passion fruit
- Pineapples
- Star fruit

Fruits with Healthy Fats

- Avocados
- Coconuts
- Olives

Oils

- Olive oil
- Coconut oil
- Cold-pressed canola oil
- Sesame oil (for flavouring)

Nut Oils (for salads and cooking)

- Almond oil
- Hazelnut oil

Omega-3 Oils (to be used cold)

- Flaxseed oil
- Hemp oil

(continued)

BodyWise Shopping List (*cont.*)

Spices/Baking Items (The sky's the limit! But for health, don't miss ...)

- Bay leaves
- Black pepper
- Cardamom
- Cayenne pepper
- Cinnamon
- Cloves
- Coriander

- Cumin
- Fennel
- Garlic
- Ginger
- Nutmeg
- Oregano
- Paprika

- Rosemary
- Saffron
- Sage
- Smoked paprika
- Thyme
- Turmeric

Classic Spice Mixes

- Chilli powder
- Chinese five-spice
- Curry powder

- Garam masala
- Herbes de Provence
- Pumpkin pie mix

- Ras el hanout
- Za'atar seasoning blend

Vinegars

- Apple cider
- Balsamic (both regular and white)

- Champagne
- Malt

- Rice
- White (grain)

Canned/Boxed Items (Be sure cans are BPA-free.)

- 'Baked' crisps (in limited quantity)
- Canned beans
- Coconut milk
- Fruit-sweetened jams

- Healthy soups
- Kale or other vegetable 'crisps' (not fried)
- Nut butters (almond, peanut, cashew, etc.)

- Pickles without sugar
- Salsa
- Seaweed snacks
- Soup stocks
- Tomato sauce

Grains

- Barley
- Bulgur
- Farro

- Wholegrain hot and cold cereals (without sugar)
- Wholegrain pasta

- Wholegrain wheat, rye, or oat breads
- Wholegrain wheat, rye, or oat crackers

Gluten-Free Grains

- Brown rice
- Coconut or potato flour
- Corn tortillas or pasta
- Oats

- Polenta or other cornmeal
- Popcorn (not microwave)

- Quinoa, millet, buckwheat, teff, tapioca, and amaranth
- Gluten-free breads and crackers

Vegetable Proteins and Dips

- Dairy free spread
- Edamame dips
- Hummus

- Muhammara
- Seitan (wheat gluten)

- Soy (non-GMO)
  edamame
  hummus
  miso
  burgers (organic)
  tempeh
  tofu

Frozen Foods

- Fruits
- Vegetables

Healthy Packaged Foods That Meet BodyWise Criteria
(Check the label.)

Treats

- Dairy-free coconut-based ice creams sweetened with agave
- Organic dark chocolate
- 'Puddings' made from avocado or silken tofu with raw cacao and sweeteners (see Appendix A)

- Sugar-free chocolate sweetened with stevia, erythritol, or both
- Wholegrain baked goods with natural sweeteners (in small quantities)

- Wholegrain gluten-free baked goods with natural sweeteners (in small quantities)

Condiments

- Bragg's Liquid Aminos
- Fish sauce
- Hot sauce

- Ketchup (agave sweetened, if possible)
- Mustards

- Nutritional yeast (brewer's yeast)
- Rice wine
- Soy sauce

Bulk Items

- Almond meal
- Beans
  black
  chickpeas (garbanzos)
  navy
  pinto
  soy
  white
- Dried fruit
- Grains

- Nuts
  almonds
  Brazil nuts
  cashews
  hazelnuts
  macadamia nuts
  peanuts
  pecans
  pine nuts
  pistachios
  walnuts

- Raw cacao powder (chocolate)
- Wholegrain flours
- Wholegrain mixes (pancakes, muffins, etc.)

(continued)

BodyWise Shopping List (*cont.*)

Meat, Fish, and Eggs

- Canned Pacific sardines or salmon (no tuna)
- Organic chicken and turkey
- Organic eggs
- Organic pork, grass-fed beef or bison, or wild game (in limited quantities)
- Organic sliced meats (without nitrates)
- Sausages
- Sustainable fish on the low-mercury list (tilapia, Pacific wild salmon, etc.)

Drinks

- Coconut kefir
- Coffee (be sure decaf is water processed)
- Herbal teas
- Kombucha
- Sparkling waters
- Teas (with decreasing levels of caffeine)
  black
  green (including matcha)
  oolong
  white
- Yerba mate (Brazilian herbal caffeinated beverage)

Coffee, Tea, and Alcohol

- Coffee, tea, or yerba mate can be healthy parts of your diet, as long as you are not having more than 2 cups of caffeinated coffee or 4 cups of black tea or yerba mate daily. If you have issues with anxiety or insomnia, it is best to avoid coffee and black tea altogether. Substituting water-processed decaffeinated coffee is an option if you love coffee but need to decrease the caffeine. For the purposes of this programme, I would recommend no more than the equivalent of 1 cup of caffeinated coffee daily, or 2 cups of black tea, or 4 cups of green tea. And all caffeine should be consumed before 2:00 p.m., depending on your sensitivity.

- Green or white tea can be enjoyed by almost everyone, unless you are very sensitive to caffeine or have significant adrenal fatigue (see Chapter 3). These teas are anti-inflammatory and prevent cancer. Green tea also increases metabolism and weight loss. As with all forms of caffeine, it should be consumed before 2:00 p.m.

- It would be ideal to eliminate alcohol altogether while doing your 28-day programme. Alcohol has a high sugar content, requires liver detoxification, and disturbs sleep patterns. However, if this one requirement keeps you from doing the programme and your body is clear that alcohol is not an addictive issue for you, you can continue to drink one drink – 340ml beer, 175ml wine, or 1 shot (45ml) spirits – three times weekly.

Special Dietary Considerations

The previous guidelines are the baseline bodywise diet, but you may want to customize your own path to health, depending on your particular health needs and goals. Here are some clues that may help you to create the best individualized programme for yourself.

Do You Need an Anti-Inflammatory Diet?

The Basic BodyWise Eating Plan is itself anti-inflammatory, but you may want to up your anti-inflammatory game, if you are at risk of or have had arthritis, cancer, or cardiovascular disease. In addition, you may want to consider increasing the anti-inflammatory part of your diet if you had:

QUIZ SCORES

Chronic Pain score of 11 or higher

Allergies and Autoimmune score of 9 or higher

Either Depression or Anxiety score of 9 or higher

Follow the chart overleaf, avoiding inflammatory foods and adding the anti-inflammatory foods and supplements suggested.

Do You Need a Low-Allergen Diet?

You may want to consider doing a low-allergen diet, also called an elimination diet, if you know or suspect that you have food sensitivities or allergies, ongoing digestive issues, or abdominal pain, or had:

QUIZ SCORES

Allergies and Autoimmune score of 9 or higher

Chronic Pain score of 16 or higher

Adding the Anti-Allergen Eating Plan

In addition to the foods you will be eliminating in the Anti-Allergen Eating plan, if you *know* that you are sensitive or allergic to a food or food group – either by testing or by your bodywise knowledge – also avoid that food or food group during your 28-day plan. People can be sensitive to a wide variety of foods, but the most common food allergies and intolerances are with cow dairy, wheat and gluten, eggs, soy, and peanuts. Other allergies and intolerances that I see in my practice involve citrus, strawberries, shellfish, tree nuts

ANTI-INFLAMMATORY EATING PLAN	
YOU WANT TO REMOVE	**YOU WANT TO PUT IN**
Inflammatory foods (avoid these altogether): fried foods, hydrogenated oils, beef, pork, cow dairy, foods that increase blood sugar (sugar, corn syrup, white flour, white rice, processed corn), processed foods	**Anti-inflammatory foods:** Aim for nine or more servings daily. One serving equals 150g of raw vegetables or fruit, 75g cooked vegetables, or 300g of raw leafy greens.
If you have arthritis: Consider eliminating nightshades, like aubergines, tomatoes, tomatillos, all peppers, and white potatoes.	**Yellow, orange, and red vegetables:** peppers, carrots, winter squash, sweet potatoes, and yams
	Dark-coloured fruits: berries, citrus, cherries, and Red Delicious and Granny Smith apples
	Dark, leafy greens: spinach, kale, and chard
	Spices: ginger, rosemary, turmeric (or curcumin), oregano, cayenne, clove, and nutmeg. Consider a supplement with turmeric (curcumin), ginger, green tea, boswellia, and/or quercetin.
	Vegetables: onions and garlic
	Beans: red kidney, pinto, and black beans
	Omega-3 fatty acids: fatty fish (wild salmon, sardines, herring), nuts (especially walnuts), flaxseed, chia seeds, hemp seeds, and leafy greens. Consider a high-quality fish-oil supplement with omega-3s EPA and DHA, with a combined amount of at least 1,500 milligrams.
	Tea: black, oolong, pu-erh, and green

(all nuts but peanuts, which are legumes), and corn. For your purposes here, you will avoid the most common five food allergens. If you feel that you might also react to citrus, strawberries, shellfish, or tree nuts, you can avoid one or all of those as well. I personally find it challenging to be off the first five, and I'd like you to be able to complete the elimination diet, so only take on as many dietary avoidances as you can practically handle! Also, if you have already eliminated gluten or dairy, say, and it has made no difference in your symptoms, you can leave it in for the purposes of this section and simply avoid the foods you haven't yet tried to stop eating.

The chart opposite lists both the common food allergens and also food

Common Food Culprits for Food Allergy and Food Intolerance

FOOD ALLERGY*

Citrus

Dairy products

Eggs

Fish

Gluten (barley, oats, rye, wheat)

Peanuts

Soy

Shellfish

Tree nuts (almonds, pecans, walnuts)

FOOD INTOLERANCE

All of the foods listed above for food allergy, plus:

Beef products

Corn

FOOD ADDITIVES

Antioxidants (butylated hydroxyanisole, butylated hydroxytoluene)

Aspartame (NutraSweet)

Biogenic amines (histamines, tyramine, octopamine, phenylethylamine)

Disaccharides (lactose)

Flavour enhancers (monosodium glutamate)

Food colours (tartrazine and various other food colours and preservatives flagged up by the Food Standards Agency)

Foods high in nickel and salicylates

Nitrates and nitrites (found in preserved meats)

Preservatives (sulphites, benzoates, and sorbates)

Refined sugars

Thickeners/stabilizers (tragacanth, agar-agar)

*The foods listed here account for roughly 80 per cent of all food hypersensitivity reactions.

From *Integrative Medicine* (textbook). ed. David Rakel, copyright 2007, 2003 by Saunders, p. 947.

additives that people often react to. You will find that, by avoiding processed food and only eating at high-quality restaurants or, preferably, at home, you can also avoid most food additives. You may want to look for these food additives in the foods you routinely consume during your 28-day plan.

AVOID THESE ALLERGENIC FOODS

Cow dairy

Eggs

Peanuts

Soy

Wheat and gluten

Comprehensive Elimination Diet Guidelines

FOODS TO INCLUDE

Animal protein: fresh or water-packed fish, wild game, lamb, duck, and organic chicken and turkey

Condiments: vinegar and all spices

Dairy substitutes: rice, oat, and nut milks, such as almond milk and coconut milk

Drinks: filtered or distilled water, decaffeinated herbal teas, and soda or mineral water

Fruits: whole fruits; unsweetened, frozen, or water-packed canned fruits; and diluted juices

Non-gluten grains and starches: brown rice, oats, millet, quinoa, amaranth, teff, tapioca, buckwheat, and coconut and potato flour

Nuts and seeds: walnuts, sesame seeds, pumpkin seeds, sunflower seeds, hazelnuts, pecans, almonds, cashews, tahini, and nut butters such as almond butter

Oils: cold-pressed olive, flax, safflower, sesame, almond, sunflower, walnut, canola, and pumpkin

Sweeteners: brown rice syrup, agave nectar, stevia, fruit sweetener, and blackstrap molasses

Vegetable protein: split peas, lentils, and legumes

Vegetables: all raw, steamed, sautéed, juiced, and roasted vegetables

FOODS TO EXCLUDE

Condiments: ketchup, relish, chutney, soy sauce, barbecue sauce, teriyaki, and other condiments that contain sugar, soy, artificial colours or preservatives

Dairy: milk, cheese, cottage cheese, cream, yogurt, butter, ice cream, frozen yogurt, and nondairy creamers

Eggs

Fats and oils: butter, margarine, shortening, processed oils, salad dressings, mayonnaise, and spreads

Grains: wheat, corn, barley, spelt, kamut, rye, and triticale

Meat: preserved meats, cold cuts, canned meats, and hot dogs with nitrates, sugar, or artificial colours

Peanuts and peanut butter

Shellfish

Soybean products: soy sauce, soybean oil in processed foods, tempeh, tofu, soy milk, soy yogurt, and textured vegetable protein

Excerpted from the Institute of Functional Medicine, introductory course materials, 2008.

Note that many processed foods, and the ingredients in them, contain forms of the allergenic foods. The following list helps you identify some of these.

IF YOU ARE AVOIDING	ALSO AVOID
Dairy	Caramel sweets, carob sweets, casein and caseinates, custard, curds, lactalbumin, goat's milk, milk chocolate, nougat, protein hydrolysate, semisweet chocolate, yogurt, pudding, whey. Also beware of flavourings: brown sugar, butter, caramel, coconut cream, 'natural flavouring,' and Simplesse.
Eggs	Albumin, apovitellin, avidin, béarnaise sauce, eggnog, egg whites, flavoprotein, globulin, hollandaise sauce, imitation egg products, livetin, lysozyme, mayonnaise, meringue, ovalbumin, ovoglycoprotein, ovomucin, ovomucoid, Simplesse
Peanuts	Egg rolls, 'high-protein' hydrolysed plant protein, hydrolysed vegetable protein, marzipan, nougat, sweets, cheesecake crusts, chilli, chocolates, sauces
Soy	Ketjap, metiauza, miso, natto, soy flour, soy protein concentrates, soy protein shakes, soy sauce, soybean hydrolysates, taotjo, tempeh, textured soy protein, textured vegetable protein, tofu, whey-soy drink. Also beware of hydrolysed plant protein, hydrolysed soy protein, hydrolysed vegetable protein, natural flavouring, vegetable broth, vegetable gum, and vegetable starch.
Wheat	Atta, bal ahar, bread flour, bulgur, cake flour, cereal extract, couscous, cracked wheat, durum flour, farina, gluten, graham flour, high-gluten flour, high-protein flour, kamut flour, malted cereals, multi-grain products, purified wheat, red wheat flakes, rolled wheat, semolina, shredded wheat, soft wheat flour, spelt, superamine, triticale, vital gluten, Vitalia macaroni, wheat protein powder, wheat starch, wheat tempeh, white flour, and wholewheat berries. Also beware of gelatinized starch, hydrolysed vegetable protein, modified food starch, starch, vegetable gum, and vegetable starch.

Modified from Joneja JV: *Dietary Management of Food Allergy and Intolerance, 2nd ed.* Hall Publishing Group, 1998; and Mahan LK, Escot-Stump S: *Food Nutrition and Diet Therapy, 11th ed.* Philadelphia, WB Saunders, 2004.

Do You Need to Detoxify?

You may want to consider adding detoxification to your 28-day programme goals if you have or have had cancer, chronic fatigue, fibromyalgia, or multiple chemical sensitivity, or had:

QUIZ SCORES

Exhaustion score of 16 or higher

Chronic Pain score of 16 or higher

Libido score of less than 11

As best you can, begin to avoid the environmental toxins listed in Chapter 3, on page 66. And as a part of your Detoxification Plan, avoid alcohol and coffee as well.

Improve Detox with Supplement Assistance

Consider supporting your liver-detox process with supplements that support liver detoxification. In addition, sweating, whether from exercise, a sauna, or the fact that it's summer, helps the body detoxify. Be sure to drink lots of water to keep up with your sweating and flush the toxins out of your system. Consider daily or twice daily dosages of the following:

NAC (N-acetyl cysteine): 100 to 300 milligrams

Glycine: 100 to 300 milligrams

Glutamine: 100 to 300 milligrams

Alpha lipoic acid: 100 to 200 milligrams

Milk thistle: 200 milligrams

Green tea extract: 25 milligrams

Do You Need Nutritional Supplementation?

You may want to add nutritional supplementation if you have a restricted diet due to food intolerances or personal preferences (i.e., vegan, Paleo, raw, avoiding many foods), or had:

QUIZ SCORES

Fatigue score of 11 or higher

Chronic Pain score of 16 or higher

Either Depression or Anxiety score of 11 or higher

Adding Nutritional Supplementation to Your Eating Plan

High-quality multivitamin with a good B-complex. Look for a reputable manufacturer who does outside testing to verify content and purity (consumerlab.com). You will also want to avoid fillers that contain gluten or lactose, as are present in many pharmacy brands, if you are sensitive or allergic. Look for levels of all of the B vitamins at 300 to 1,000 per cent over the RDA (recommended dietary allowance), as some of us need higher doses because of our genetics and environmental stressors. Also, if depression is an issue, you may want to do a methylated form of folic acid and B_{12} (discussed in Chapter 6). When you look at B_{12}, it should say methylcobalamin rather than cyanocobalamin. Instead of folic acid, it should have methyl-tetrahydrofolate (MTHF). And for treating depression, you will want at least 2 milligrams of MTHF and 1 milligram of methyl B_{12}. It may make sense to take a multivitamin and add the methylated B vitamins separately. They are available individually or as part of a B complex. Note that food-based multivitamins are probably absorbed better, but tend to have lower amounts of vitamin content. If you have issues with anxiety, insomnia, palpitations, or muscle pain, you may also want to add an absorbable form of magnesium, such as magnesium glycinate, aspartate, or amino acid chelate at a dose of 200 to 500 milligrams. Keep in mind that high doses of magnesium can cause diarrhoea, so back off it if this is the case for you. If constipation is an issue, magnesium citrate or oxide can also be useful to loosen stools.

Vitamin D_3. I would strongly recommend that you test your vitamin D levels to see whether you truly need vitamin D, but taking 10mg/day is sufficient for most. Some of my patients are so deficient and have such poor absorption that they need much higher doses. However, higher doses are not safe to take unless you measure your levels, as vitamin D is fat soluble and will build up in the body to toxic levels if too much is taken.

Fish oil. The omega-3 fatty acids in fish oil have been shown to reduce triglycerides, improve inflammation (think arthritis, allergy, and auto-immune disease), and may reduce anxiety and depression. If you have any of these conditions, taking a quality fish-oil supplement may be helpful. I would recommend a brand that is outside-tested for contaminants and is consistent with European standards for contaminants because Europe has stricter standards than the United States. You also want a brand that is tested for shelf-life and has an expiry date. For the conditions above, I recommend looking at the omega-3 content of the fish oil, and the EPA and DHA portions, both of which are important. You want to take an oil or a number of capsules equivalent to 1,000 to 1,500 milligrams of EPA and DHA.

Antidepressant herbs/supplements. If depression is an ongoing issue, you may want to consider any of the herbs and/or supplements that we discussed in Chapter 6. Please consult that chapter for risks and benefits as well as potential interactions with other medications.

Checking In on Your BodyWise Eating Plan for the Next 3 Weeks

After Week 1

How did your 1st week go? Do you feel any different eating this way? Continue with the Basic BodyWise Eating Plan and any additional programmes that you chose to add to your plan during Week 2 as well. If you are doing an elimination diet, hang tight! You will start adding foods back to your diet in Week 3.

After Week 2

If you chose to do the low-allergen plan with the elimination diet, now is the time to begin to experiment with your diet. First of all, how do you feel now in comparison with when you started? Any change in energy? Pain? Digestion or abdominal pain? Mood? This week, I want you to begin to introduce the allergenic foods that you have taken out, one at a time. You can do this in any order that you desire, but I would recommend putting the foods you are most concerned about in first. For example, if you suspect you are gluten sensitive, add gluten back to your diet for the next 3 days. Is there any change in how you feel? You'll want to keep track of this on the chart below. After 3 days of eating gluten, take it back out again. Then add your next food, for example, cow dairy, and eat it for 3 days. In this way, continue to add a new food for 3 days, noting reactions, and then taking it out again. If you eliminated just the five most allergenic foods, you should complete this process of introducing foods on your 29th day. If you eliminated other foods, it will take a bit longer. What you do with the information you gathered with your elimination diet is up to you. Some of my patients have quite dramatic reactions to eating certain foods and are happy to keep those out

ELIMINATION DIET	DAY 1	DAY 2	DAY 3	DAY 4	DAY 5	DAY 6
Breakfast						
Reactions?						
Lunch						
Reactions?						
Dinner						
Reactions?						

of their diets to feel better. Other patients have milder reactions and simply limit the food in question, or eat it infrequently.

After Week 3

How does your body feel compared to when you started your plan? Keep it going for another week. And if you are doing the anti-allergen eating plan, keep adding foods back in this week and noting how you feel when you eat them.

After Week 4

You can continue any eating habits that you know have been helpful for you, as every dietary recommendation is safe to continue long-term, if you'd like. If you completed the low-allergen add-on with the elimination diet, you should continue adding additional foods until you've tried all of them and got a sense of whether they affect your health and well-being. It's fine to add back any eliminated foods that your body feels fine with. If you had some negative reactions to food groups, you may want to keep them out of your diet, or add them back, but in limited quantity. It's also worth noting that some of my patients can eat gluten in the form of rye, or barley, but not wheat. Continue to explore what works best in your body.

Week 2: Sleep, Rest, and Rejuvenation

This week is your opportunity to feel rested and refreshed. Remember what that was like? Whatever your sleep habits are now, you are hoping to shift them just a bit in a direction that will impact your vitality and well-being.

Your goal is to wake up in the morning feeling rested and ready to get out of bed. For a select few, this happens after 6.5 to 7 hours of sleep. But for the great majority, this occurs after at least 8 hours of good-quality sleep. For the purposes of this week of the programme, see if you can manage to preserve at least 8 hours of time to sleep each night.

If you have a device to track sleep cycles, you can use it this week to get feedback on your sleep. Either on your phone or computer, or right here in the book, track your sleep for this week using the chart on pages 226 to 227.

Step 1: Commit to sleeping at least 8 hours each night for the next 3 weeks.

Get out your calendar and plan your days so that you are finished with your tasks and have the time you need to get ready for bed and to fall asleep, and still guarantee 8 hours. If you wake up naturally very early, or you rise early for work or other responsibilities, you will need to go to bed early as well. When will you need to eat, leave work, and so on in order to get to bed on time? If you sleep with another person, you will want to discuss this with him and, ideally, get his support. Put a note on your mirror that says 'Go to bed' if you have to.

Step 2: Remove any barriers that interfere with your sleep.

If you have trouble falling asleep:

- Eliminate caffeine completely or cut back to the equivalent of 1 cup of coffee or 2 cups of black tea per day. And make sure you have your caffeine before noon.
- Avoid medications that interfere with sleep if at all possible (see the list on page 156). But please don't stop prescription medications without checking with your doctor.

TIME	SUN	MON	TUES
In bed at	11:15 p.m.	10:45	11:00
Sleep onset	12:00	11:00	11:15
Any awakening(s) at night? How long?	Once for 15 minutes to pee	Once for 25 minutes at 2:00 a.m.	Up at 2:30–4:00 a.m. (stressed about project)
Awake in a.m.	6:30	6:30	6:30
Sleep hours	6 hours, 15 minutes	7 hours, 5 minutes	5 hours, 45 minutes
Quality of sleep	Good	Okay	Lousy
Any sleep strategies used (behaviours, herbs, etc.)?	Bath and herbal tea before bed	Valerian root, 200 milligrams	Too anxious, on computer before bed and in middle of night
Any alcohol or caffeine during the day before?	Cup of coffee at 10:00 a.m. and 2:30 p.m.	Cup of coffee at 10:00 a.m. and 2:30 p.m.	Cup of coffee at 7:00 and 10:00 a.m., and 1:00 p.m.
How did you feel in the morning?	Tired when the alarm went off	Tired	Awful, headache, nauseated

- Avoid LED screens for at least 2 hours before sleep. And consider adding an app to your phone or computer that dims the blue light exposure of your phone, pad, or computer (justgetflux.com), especially if it is impossible to avoid screens for 2 hours before sleep. If you must watch television, do it on a television screen, not a computer, and be sure that the screen is at least 4 feet from your eyes. This will limit the amount of light from the television that stimulates your brain.

Step 3: Nurture your sleep.

To help ready you for sleep:

- Have a small snack before bed that is a combination of a complex carbohydrate and a protein (a small slice of turkey and/or cheese on a wholegrain cracker or slice of apple).
- Consider a hot shower or bath before bed.
- Try to make your bedroom dark, cool, quiet, and free of electronic devices (this means your mobile phone).

WED	THURS	FRI	SAT
10:00	10:15	11:30	Midnight
Fast	10:30	Fast	Fast
Up at 3:00 a.m. to pee, 20 minutes to fall back to sleep	Siren woke me up at 2:00 a.m. Took L-theanine and did deep breathing. Back to sleep by 2:30.	None	Up to pee at 3:00 a.m., and up until 3:45
6:30	6:30	8:30	9:00
8 hours, 10 minutes	7 hours, 30 minutes	9 hours	8 hours, 15 minutes
Good	Good	Great	Okay
Valerian root, 400 milligrams, no screens after 9:00 p.m.	Valerian root, 400 milligrams, no screens after 8:30 p.m.	Valerian root, 400 milligrams	Valerian root, 400 milligrams
Black tea in morning and at lunch	Half decaf coffee for breakfast, black tea at lunch	Black tea at breakfast and lunch	2 glasses of wine before bed
Better, a little tired	Tired, otherwise good	Good!	A little foggy, headache

TIME	SUN	MON	TUES
In bed at			
Sleep onset			
Any awakening(s) at night? How long?			
Awake in a.m.			
Sleep hours			
Quality of sleep			
Any sleep strategies used (behaviours, herbs, etc.)?			
Any alcohol or caffeine during the day before?			
How did you feel in the morning?			

If you have trouble staying asleep:

- Consider finding other sleep arrangements for a sleep-disturbing pet or child.
- Use earplugs, if needed, for a snoring or noisy partner or roommate.
- Consider valerian root, passionflower, magnesium, 5-HTP, or melatonin to help you go to sleep.
- Avoid alcohol after 6:00 p.m., as it can lead to middle-of-the-night awakening.
- If you are perimenopausal or menopausal with hot flushes that disturb sleep, consider seeing your doctor for treatment.
- Use meditative practices for falling back asleep. The belly breathing exercise (page 21) and body awareness exercise (page 30) are great for this. During the body awareness exercise, imagine that each part of your body is relaxing and becoming heavy and warm as you breathe into it.
- Consider L-theanine at 100 to 200 milligrams, or Lavela (micronized lavender oil) to help calm the mind and put you back to sleep.

WED	THURS	FRI	SAT

Consider which of these recommendations are most relevant for your sleep cycle and make your 'sleep plan' for the week. Make a commitment to your bedtime, and plan your afternoon and evening as best you can to reach your bed in time to get enough sleep.

Checking In on Your Bodywise Sleeping Plan in the Next 3 Weeks

How did you feel at the end of Week 2 after trying to have more sleep with better sleep quality? Typically, it takes some time to determine the optimal sleep regime for yourself. Stay committed to trying to sleep at least 8 hours per night through the rest of the 28-day programme. It will make all of the other changes more effective. In fact, getting enough sleep has a profound effect on weight loss, if that is something you desire. You can continue to track your sleep on the chart on pages 230 to 231, if you would like.

If exhaustion is a significant complaint of yours and after a few weeks you are still not sleeping well, be sure you are using all the tools from the sleep chapter. And if you haven't yet tried any of the herbs or supplements for sleep, now may be the time to do so. If sleep continues to elude you, a sleep study or visit to your doctor may be important for finding a solution. Sleeping well is vital to your health and vitality.

Week 3: Move

This week, you get to focus on moving your body in a way that helps you be healthier, stronger, and more flexible. It is vital that you are bodywise in selecting an activity and a level of exertion that are friendly to your body. Close your eyes, take a deep breath, and sense what movement your body may be longing for. Hiking in nature? Riding a bike? Dancing with your girlfriends? Tai chi in the park? Or, perhaps your body is longing to crawl into bed for a nap? All movement is therapeutic. Maybe walk the long way to your bed. Finding some activity that you long for and love is vital to your success in bodywise movement.

Certain exercises, such as gentle yoga, Pilates, tai chi, or qigong, can be therapeutic and also adapted to different levels of ability. Yoga can be wonderful for extending the spine and increasing flexibility in women with neck and back pain. Pilates can build core strength that prevents injuries of the neck, back, shoulders, and hips. Tai chi and qigong help develop smooth flow of the joints and alignment that fosters painless, fluid movement. Swimming and water aerobics are terrific workouts for those who experience pain with bearing weight, such as arthritis of the feet, knees, hips, and spine. What movement might be therapeutic in supporting your body to be as vital as possible?

Consider the Three Aspects of Fitness

How is your aerobic capacity? Aerobic exercise is literally movement that makes you breathe hard. Climbing stairs, hiking, and riding a bike are all examples of this. A healthy woman, at any age, if she isn't injured, should be able to climb at least a flight of stairs without getting winded. And all of us need aerobic exercise of some kind. My patient Beverly is 72 and gardens extensively in her yard. This involves lifting, digging, and pulling weeds – mostly strength-building activities. We agreed that she needed to complement her gardening, which she loves, with some more aerobic exercise. She decided to walk around her neighbourhood for 30 minutes 4 days a week, in addition to her gardening. If you feel that you need to work on this, any of the activities that require ongoing movement and increased breath rate work: dancing, walking, running, cycling, swimming, various aerobic 'machines' at the gym, or sports that include running, swimming, or jumping (i.e., netball, football, volleyball, tennis).

How is your strength? Do you need to strengthen your body? Strength helps us to carry groceries, get up and down off the floor with ease, or lift furniture. Strength-building is especially important as we get older since it helps to maintain muscle mass and bone density and prevents injury. Getting some direction on form is essential to strength-building, whether you are doing squats or using free weights or machines. Most gyms have personnel or a trainer who can help you get started, or you can watch yourself performing a move in the mirror and match it to the form of a professional image that you see online or in a book. If you want to do a simple home workout, checking out online videos on how to combine simple exercises, such as squats, jumping exercises, push-ups, and forms of sit-ups to increase overall muscle tone can work wonders. I give a few examples in Chapter 10.

How is your flexibility? Interestingly, you can be aerobically fit and strong, but lack balance and flexibility, making you more vulnerable to injury. Simple stretching before or after exercise can be beneficial for keeping your body moving. Yoga, martial arts, and dance are all wonderful forms that increase both balance and flexibility. And you'd be surprised how much increasing the flexibility of your body can increase the flexibility of your thoughts as well!

What kinds of movement do you need to add to your life to enhance your well-being? At a minimum, most of us need 150 minutes weekly of some form of moderate exercise (and walking counts!). Recall that moderate exercise gets your heart rate into the 50th to 75th percentile, as discussed in Chapter 10. You can check the chart on page 172 to calculate your target heart rate. If you are not yet exercising for 150 minutes weekly, then that should be your goal for this week. Remember that walking at your lunch break or breaking up the walking into different parts of the day counts. One of my patients has counted off the steps between her desk and the far conference room at work and tries to make the trip at least three times daily during her work rounds. What is a realistic goal that you can set for yourself? If you have an electronic device that counts steps (your phone or a wristband or watch), see if you can get in 10,000 steps at least 3 days a week. If your exercise routine already easily meets these goals, what else can you set in place to balance your fitness? Might you add a class or 30-minute-plus workout video to your routine once per week? Or a strength routine? Or, perhaps you want to try the high-intensity interval training (HIIT) described in Chapter 10 to increase muscle mass and longevity? Listen to your body as you choose and experience your movement routine.

	DAY 1	DAY 2	DAY 3
Type of exercise			
Time or number of steps			
How did you feel before and after?			

Enhance and alter your movement as you go, to fit your body's needs. If you had a rough night, and you're exhausted, it may not be the day for your HIIT workout. An online yoga class may be a better fit. The goal is not a particular number of steps walked or calories burned, but to listen to your body and find ways to move every single day that engage and awaken your physical power and enjoyment.

Design this week's fitness plan according to your needs and desires using the table on this page.

When deciding where to focus the first step of your movement journey, consider how your scores on the chapter quizzes may also inform your exercise choices.

If your Fatigue score is 16 or above: Some amount of activity is important no matter what your level of fatigue, but you need to listen closely to your body's needs when choosing how long to exert yourself. You will want to be careful about overexerting yourself, as it can increase your overall exhaustion or cause injury. I love the therapeutic quality of gentle yoga (Hatha, Anusara, or restorative yoga). When fatigue is a significant issue, I would not recommend any kind of 'hot yoga.' Though it is a workout and detoxifying, it is also depleting, in that you sweat out your minerals and the heat can exacerbate fatigue. I love tai chi and qigong for their ability to reenergize you with qi, or vital energy – so important for someone with significant fatigue. Walking or gentle water aerobics would be other options.

If your Chronic Pain score is 11 or above: You will definitely want to consider your vulnerabilities or injuries in designing your movement programme. Seeing a physiotherapist can be very helpful for increasing strength, reducing pain, and designing an exercise programme for your future wellness. Keep in mind that physiotherapists, like all practitioners, have differing levels of skill and expertise. It is worth finding someone that you really like and respect and who understands your body. In addition, you may find

DAY 4	DAY 5	DAY 6	DAY 7

a hands-on practitioner – chiropractor, osteopath, or massage therapist – that helps keep your body in alignment and able to move painlessly.

If your Libido score is less than 11: Great news: Regular aerobic exercise increases libido! Getting in at least 30 minutes of aerobic exercise at least 3 days a week will stoke your sex life; in part, because exercise helps you feel more *in* your body and gets your blood flowing. There is really nothing better for sex drive than exercise that gets your pelvis moving. Something like Zumba, salsa dancing, African dancing, hula, belly dancing, samba, or tango can get the blood flowing in a way that lights up your cheeks and your pelvic area. Women in more northern cultures tend to do activities that are in a straight line (walking, running, swimming, cycling, etc.) and developing the ability to swing your hips from side to side with precision is a beautiful and ancient female art that can get the juices flowing.

If your Depression or Anxiety score is 11 or higher: It is vital for you to have a regular exercise routine. As discussed in Chapter 6, regular exercise is *more* effective in treating long-term depression than medication. And exercise is a potent treatment for anxiety as well. Most of these studies looked at the effects of aerobic exercise. I recommend that my patients with depression and anxiety do some form of aerobic activity for at least 30 minutes 5 days a week. It is particularly effective if that activity can happen outside, given the therapeutic effect of sunlight, vitamin D absorption, and nature. If anxiety is your major symptom, exercise that is calming and meditative, such as yoga, tai chi, or qigong, can also be of benefit.

Week 4: Cultivating Love, Community, and Purpose

Close your eyes and take a deep breath. Put your fingertips on your heart and continue to breathe deeply, as if you are breathing right into your heart itself. As you breathe, feel your heart soften and begin to open, like a rose, petal by petal. Ask your heart the questions:

'What kind of love do I need in my life?'

'What kind of people would I like to be closer to?'

'How can I make that happen?'

Consider your answers and write them down in this book or in a journal, if you would like. What is one action you could take this week to increase love and community in your life? More hugs from your friends? A massage? Get on the dating site you've been meaning to pursue? Schedule a date with your partner? If your score on the Social Network Index (see page 183) was 3 or less, you may want to concentrate on broadening your community. If your score on the Depression or Anxiety quiz was 11 or higher, this section is particularly important for you, as relationships and community heal our suffering hearts.

Choose two actions to take this week to enhance your love experience.

1. _____

_____

2. _____

_____

In Chapter 12, we focused on finding a sense of purpose – doing something in the world for others that gives you a sense of meaning. Your purpose doesn't need to be fancy or far-reaching. It simply helps you feel needed and reminds you why you are here. Which is vital for your health.

If you haven't already, do the three-step exercise on pages 194 to 199 that helps you arrive at an aspect of your purpose, your particular work in the world. Choose one of the ideas that you found that feels in alignment with your sense of purpose. One that calls to you at this moment. An idea that, when you contemplate it, makes your body say 'yes!' (You may want to revisit 'Exercise 1: Tuning in to Your "Yes" and "No"' on page 9.) Think of one concrete action that you can take this week to bring this sense of purpose into your reality. For example, you could volunteer to organize charity work in your workplace. You could sign up for a class in a skill that gives you pleasure. You could explore the possibility of further schooling or training that will allow you to do work that you love. You could find a moment in your current work when you reach out to a customer or colleague with compassion. First steps are just that, first steps. So this week, simply make the first phone call or have the conversation or explore the financial options – whatever first steps will lead you toward your goal. Whatever you choose, be sure that you can take this step this week.

Action step toward my purpose: _____

_____

Completing Your BodyWise 28-Day Plan!

Congratulations! Four weeks is a long time to commit to yourself, and you did it! If you are like me or any other normal human, you probably had a few slips along the way. I want to be clear that doing it perfectly is not the point here. Take a deep breath and appreciate yourself for any small change that you *did* make this month. Forgive the rest, and let it go.

The most important part of this programme is to gain a better sense of your bodywise wisdom in action. What choices and changes did you make this month that your body liked? How did you feel when you made them? How can you keep some of those going? The BodyWise Plan can be a guideline for your choices long after you finish your 'plan.' It is a healthy, long-term way of eating, moving, and living that, when combined with your own intuition about what your body needs, can give you years of healing and vitality. Keep reaching for more ways to receive and give love in the world. Your heart is your finest healer.

Helpful Information

Measuring Waist and Hip Circumference

Waist circumference: Feel your lowest rib (the 10th rib). Then feel the top of your hip bone in the front, and split the difference. This middle zone is where you want to measure your waist – halfway between your 10th rib and hip bone. From behind, wrap the tape measure around your waist and note the measurement.

Hip circumference: Find the head of your thighbone (the greater trochanter)

How Do You Measure Waist-to-Hip Ratio?

Use an ordinary tape measure and:

- Measure your waist at its narrowest (usually at the belly button or just above it)
- Measure your hips at the widest part, around your buttocks.

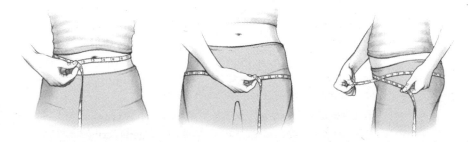

where it sticks out on the side of your thigh in your hip area. Measure over the top of your greater trochanters for hip circumference.

The waist-to-hip ratio can predict cardiovascular risk. Your waist measurement divided by your hip measurement is ideally less than or equal to 0.8 inch as a woman. In a man, we want it less than or equal to 1 inch. A higher ratio means a higher risk.

How to Choose Safe and Effective Supplements

Supplements, unlike medications, are not regulated by the MHRA, and therefore vary tremendously in quality and quantity of content. You will want to ask a knowledgeable person at the shop if there are brands available that have outside testing agencies verify their content. Four testing agencies are listed overleaf, with their 'seals' that you can look for on products you are interested in. I'm including a summary of this information from supplementquality.com.

Avoiding Airborne Allergens
Dust Mites

Dust mite allergens are a common trigger of allergy and asthma symptoms. Dust mites are microscopic creatures that are close relatives of ticks and spiders. They feed on skin cells shed by people, and they thrive in warm, humid environments such as bedding, upholstered furniture, and carpeting.

Avoiding exposure to dust mites is the best strategy for controlling dust mite allergy. Because you spend so much time in the bedroom, it is important to focus your energy here to reduce dust mite levels. So what can you do to reduce your exposure to these little creatures? Although you will never be able to completely eliminate dust mites, here are some recommendations to reduce your exposure.

- **Use allergen-proof bed coverings:** Cover your pillows and mattress with dustproof or allergen covers. These are covers that are made of tightly woven fabric and prevent dust mites from moving in or out of your bedding. You can also encase box springs, but most important are the surfaces that you make contact with during sleep.
- **Wash bedding weekly.** Wash all sheets, blankets, pillowcases, and bed covers at 60°C to kill dust mites and remove allergens; cold or warm water won't do the trick. If bedding can't be washed in hot water, put the items in the dryer for at least 15 minutes at a temperature above 130°F.

Four Websites That List Quality Products and Companies

DECEMBER 20 2002, LINKS UPDATED JANUARY 2007
BY WYN SNOW, MANAGING EDITOR AT SUPPLEMENTQUALITY.COM

Four organizations currently perform quality testing and inspections of supplement products and/or manufacturing plants. Here are the quality seals you can expect to see on products, together with links to lists and/or databases on the corresponding websites.

consumerlab.com   Natural Products   NSF International
                         Association   (nsf.org)
                         (npainfo.org)

WHAT DO THESE QUALITY SEALS MEAN?

1. Consumerlab.com
Independent product testing: ConsumerLab examines the research literature to understand the chemical makeup of products that have been shown useful in clinical (i.e., human) research studies – and establishes standards of quality for those products. It then selects popular brands for testing against these standards, which include identity and potency, purity, bioavailability, and consistency. ConsumerLab also has programmes that test raw materials and screen supplements for substances banned by athletic organizations (in particular, the Olympics). For more information, see consumerlab.com. (You must be a subscriber to access the full lists of products that pass testing.)

2. Natural Products Association (NPA, formerly NNFA)
Manufacturing plant inspections: NNFA's GMP Certification Programme inspects manufacturing plants of member companies to determine if they are complying

with good manufacturing practices (GMPs) developed by NNFA in collaboration with several other industry trade organizations. These GMPs include standards for quality control/assurance, cleanliness, checking identity and potency of ingredients, and testing of final products for potency, purity, and bioavailability. (NNFA's GMP standards are the same as those for NSF International.) (Go to the NNFA list of certified companies.)

3. NSF International
Manufacturing plant inspections: NSF International's International Standard for Dietary Supplements uses the same set of criteria for good manufacturing practices as NNFA. NSF International convened a committee of stakeholders – including individuals from industry, government, and consumer groups – who voted on the criteria in the standard. Negative votes must be resolved before the standard is approved. As noted under NNFA, these GMP standards cover quality control/assurance, cleanliness, checking identity and potency of ingredients, and testing of final products for potency, purity, and bioavailability. While NNFA's GMP Certification Programme is available only to NNFA members, any company can apply for certification by NSF International. (Go to the NSF International database of certified companies and products. For a full list, leave the product search and manufacturer boxes blank.)

WHAT DO THESE CRITERIA MEAN?

1. Identity and potency: Does the product contain the ingredients and dosage strength listed on the label?
2. Purity: Is the product free of specific contaminants it should not have?
3. Bioavailability: Does the product dissolve adequately for use in the body?
4. Consistency: Does each tablet or other unit of the product have the same identity, potency, and purity?
5. Good manufacturing practices (GMPs): Does the manufacturing facility follow high-quality standards for
   - NPA/NSFIn'tl: procedures for quality control/assurance, cleanliness, checking identity and potency of ingredients, and testing of final products for potency, purity, and bioavailability?
   - USP: safe, sanitary, and well-controlled procedures?

You can also freeze nonwashable items, such as stuffed animals, for at least 12 hours once a month, which will kill the dust mites.

- **Keep humidity low.** Keep your home humidity below 50 per cent. A dehumidifier or air-conditioner can help keep humidity low. You can also buy a device that can measure humidity levels at your local hardware store or online.

- **Declutter and dust.** Remove clutter, especially next to your bed, to prevent the accumulation of dust. To remove dust, use a damp or oiled mop or rag rather than dry materials, to prevent the dust from becoming airborne and resettling.

- **Vacuum regularly.** Use a vacuum cleaner with a double-layered microfilter bag or a high-efficiency particulate air (HEPA) filter. If your allergies flare up when vacuuming, leave the area being vacuumed while someone else does the work. Stay out of the vacuumed room for about 2 hours after vacuuming.

- **Remove carpeting and other dust mite habitats.** Carpeting provides a comfortable and humid environment for dust mites. If possible, replace wall-to-wall bedroom carpeting with tile, wood, or laminate flooring. Consider replacing other dust-collecting furnishings in bedrooms, such as upholstered furniture, nonwashable curtains, and horizontal blinds.

- **Install a high-efficiency media filter in your boiler and air-conditioning unit.** Look for a filter with a good EPC rating (Energy Performance Certificate), and leave the fan on to create a whole-house air filter. Be sure to change the filter every 3 months.

Mould and Pollen and Animal Dander

Many of these steps were also important for dust mite avoidance above.

- **For mould allergy, keep humidity low.** Keep your home humidity below 50 per cent. A dehumidifier or air conditioner can help keep humidity low. You can also buy a device that can measure humidity levels at your local hardware store or online.

- **Consider home testing for mould spores.** You can use the do-it-yourself version or hire someone to do it for you, but identifying which moulds are present and which parts of the house they are in is key. It can be as simple as installing better bathroom ventilation and using a weak bleach solution to clean mould off of the walls, or as complex as needing to investigate behind walls or under floors for water leakage and mould growth. If moving to a sunnier, drier location is an option, sometimes that is easier.

- **De-clutter and dust.** Pollen, pet dander, and mould spores accumulate in dust. Remove clutter, especially next to your bed, to prevent the accumulation of dust. To remove dust, use a damp or oiled mop or rag rather than dry materials, to prevent the dust from becoming airborne and resettling.
- **Vacuum regularly.** Use a vacuum cleaner with a double-layered micro-filter bag or a high-efficiency particulate air (HEPA) filter. If your allergies flare up when vacuuming, leave the area being vacuumed while someone else does the work. Stay out of the vacuumed room for about 2 hours after vacuuming.
- **Remove carpeting.** It accumulates all allergens.
- **Install a high-efficiency media filter in your boiler and air conditioning unit.** Look for a filter with a good EPC rating (Energy Performance Certificate), and leave the fan on to create a whole-house air filter. Be sure to change the filter every 3 months.
- **Keep pets away.** Pets that you are allergic to should *at least* be out of your bedroom. Ideally, of course, they would remain outside the house altogether.
- **Avoid outdoor exercise.** If you are pollen-allergic, stay inside between 5:00 and 10:00 in the morning. Airborne pollen levels are typically at their highest then, especially on dry, windy days.
- **Consider purchasing a HEPA air filter.** This is a good idea for your bedroom or any indoor room you spend a lot of time in. There are many to choose from, but you are looking for one that exchanges all of the air in the room you are purchasing it for, *at least* two to three times per hour, with more being better (>2 ACH, or air changes per hour). These are useful for mould spores, animal dander, and pollen.
- **Use a neti pot.** This, or a saltwater rinse bottle, should be used regularly. There is a measurable reduction in symptoms when you rinse the allergens from your nose two or three times daily, and salt acts as a mild decongestant. You can use a neti pot with warm water and this solution: 250ml warm water, 1 teaspoon salt, and a pinch of baking soda. Or, you can buy a bottle or neti pot with pre-packaged and measured ingredients (such as Sinus Rinse).

Choosing a Probiotic

If you are interested in purchasing a probiotic for regular health maintenance, a quality, refrigerated mix of lactobacillus and bifidobacter species will do. You want to look at how many colony forming units (CFU) are present and, of course, be sure that that number is guaranteed at the time of purchase, not at the time of its manufacture. For health maintenance, 20 billion CFU will suffice. If you have ongoing digestive issues, significant allergies, or autoimmune disease, or currently have inflammatory bowel disease, much higher doses are needed to be effective. I use from 100 to 400 billion CFU in my patients to treat these disorders. If repopulating normal bacteria is challenging, I sometimes include a healthy protective fungus, *Saccharomyces boulardii*, with the probiotic supplements. It can also be helpful to use prebiotics, soluble fibre supplements that feed the healthy bacteria. And do not forget that fermented foods are wonderful sources of broader types of bacteria that help create a strong gut bacterial environment.

Raw Cacao Balls

135g almonds

3 tablespoons cacao powder, plus more for coating

1 teaspoon vanilla extract

2 tablespoons coconut oil

2–3 tablespoons agave nectar (for less sugar, instead of agave, use a combination of erythritol and stevia, or either of these mixed with agave to limit sugar calories)

3 tablespoons full-fat coconut milk

Pinch of salt

Combine all ingredients in a blender or food processor. Should be thick, like cake batter. If not, refrigerate until solid. Pull out a tablespoon or two at a time and roll into balls. Roll in cacao powder to coat and place on baking paper in the refrigerator. Enjoy when they are firm.

Possible additions:
Shredded coconut, Cayenne, Nut butter, Cinnamon, Goji berries

Chocolate Avocado Pudding
(from http://allrecipes.com/recipe/234324/chocolate-avocado-pudding/)

2 large avocados, peeled, pitted, and cubed

55g unsweetened cocoa powder

40g cup coconut sugar, or less to taste (can use a combination of stevia, erythritol, and agave to limit sugar calories)

15ml coconut milk

2 teaspoons vanilla extract

1 pinch ground cinnamon

Blend avocados, cocoa powder, coconut sugar or sugar substitutes, coconut milk, vanilla extract, and cinnamon in a blender until smooth. Refrigerate pudding until chilled, about 30 minutes.

Considerations for Hormone-Replacement Therapy

The most effective treatment we have available for hot flushes is hormone-replacement therapy with oestrogen. This is controversial for a number of reasons. Oestrogens stimulate the breasts and uterus, and excessive oestrogen exposure increases the risk of both breast and uterine cancer. Oestrogens also increase blood clotting and may predispose women to heart attacks, strokes, and blood clots. We know this because women who have had many more years of periods – with early onset of periods, no child-bearing interrupting periods, and/or late menopause – are at higher risk for oestrogen-dependent cancers. It is then not surprising that the largest study done to date on using Premarin and Provera (artificial oestrogens and progestogens) showed an increased risk of breast cancer in women on hormone-replacement therapy beyond the age of 60. Most doctors are cautious about using hormone-replacement therapy, and many are choosing to use bioidentical hormones. *Bioidentical* simply means that the hormones (unlike Premarin or Provera, which are synthetic) are identical to the hormones that our own bodies produce. Bioidentical hormones are now widely available by prescription from both regular and complementary health chemists, in patches, gels, creams, and oral tablets. The oral versions of oestrogen require liver metabolism and are more likely to cause blood clots, heart attacks, strokes, and deep-vein thrombosis or blood clot. For that reason, I always recommend that my patients use oestrogen that is absorbed through the skin – via patches, creams, gels, or vaginal suppositories.

Along with oestrogen, progesterone is required in women who have a uterus, to protect the uterus from the stimulating effect of the oestrogen therapy. In other words, without progesterone, oestrogen-replacement therapy alone can increase the risk of uterine cancer. In women who have had their uteruses removed, it is fine to use oestrogen alone for hormone replacement. There appears to be very little risk for using hormone-replacement therapy for up to 5 years around the time of menopause. There is even less risk in using oestrogen alone – in those women without a uterus – for up to 7 years after the time of menopause. The North American Menopause Society, in its 2016 recommendations, says, 'The lowest dose of hormone therapy should be used for the shortest duration needed to manage menopausal symptoms.' And most practitioners would agree with this recommendation.[1]

It is worth noting that some women, unfortunately, have hot flushes ongoing for a lifetime. And some women have such a profound positive improvement in mood and cognition with hormone-replacement therapy that they want to continue for longer. In such situations, you need to really tune in to your body; use your body intelligence to balance the potential risks with the benefits in your particular situation.

Orgasm-Inhibiting Prescription Drugs

Acebutolol (Sectral)

Alprazolam (Xanax)

Amitriptyline (Triptafen)

Anexia

Atenolol (Tenormin)

Bisoprolol (Cardicor)

Carbamazepine (Tegretol)

Carvedilol

Chlorazepate (Tranxene)

Chlordiazepoxide (Librium)

Chlorpromazine (Largactil)

Chlorprothixene (Taractan)

Citalopram (Cipramil)

Clomipramine (Anafranil)

Clonazepam (Rivotril)

Codeine (Tylenol with codeine)

Dexamphetamine (Adderall, Dexedrine, Dextrostat)

Diazepam (Valium)

Disulfiram (Antabuse)

Doxepin (Sinepin)

Escitalopram (Cipralex)

Esmolol (Brevibloc)

Ethosuximide

Fenfluramine (Emiside)

Fentanyl (Duragesic Patches, Actiq)

Fluoxetine (Prozac)

Fluphenazine (Modecate)

Flurazepam (Dalmane)

Fluvoxamine (Faverin)

Hydromorphone

Imipramine (Palladone)

Ketoconazole (Nizoral)

Labetolol (Trandate)

Lorazepam

Lorcet

Lortab

Meperidine (Demerol)

Methadone

Methylphenidate (Ritalin, Concerta)

Methyldopa (Aldomet)

Metoprolol (Lopressor)

Mexidone

Modafinil (Provigil, Alertec)

Morphine (Sevredol, Oramorph, Morphgesic, MST Continus, Zomorph)

Nadolol (Corgard)

Norco

Nortriptyline (Allegron)

Oxazepam

Oxycodone (Oxynorm, Oxycontin, Langtec)

Paroxetine (Seroxat)

Penbutolol (Levatol)

Perphenazine (Fentazin)

Pethidine

Phentermine (Adipex-P, Ionamin, Phentride, Phentercot, Teramine, Pro-Fast, Oby-Trim)

Pimozide (Orap)

Pindolol

Prochlorperazine (Stemetil)

Propoxyphene (Darvon, Darvocet, Wygesic)

Propranolol (Inderal)

Risperidone (Risperidal)

Sertraline (Lustral)

Sibutramine (Meridia)

Temazepam

Timolol (Prestim)

Trifluoperazine (Stelazine)

Trimipramine (Surmontil)

Venlafaxine (Efexor)

Zyclone

Common Drugs That Decrease Your Libido

Acebutolol (Sectral)

Acetazolamide (Diamox)

Alprazolam (Xanax)

Amiodarone (Cordarone, Pacerone)

Amitriptyline (Triptafen)

Atenolol (Tenormin)

Barbiturates (Fiorinal, butalbital)

Birth control pills

Bisoprolol (Cardicor)

Carbamazepine (Tegretol)

Carvedilol

Chlordiazepoxide (Librium)

Chlorpromazine (Largactil)

Cimetidine (Tagamet)

Clomipramine (Anafranil)

Clonazepam (Rivotril)

Diazepam (Valium)

Digoxin (Lanoxin)

Doxepin (Sinepin)

Esmolol (Brevibloc)

Ethosuximide (Emeside)

Famotidine

Fenfluramine (Pondimin)

Flurazepam

Imipramine

Interferon

Isocarboxazid (Marplan)

Ketoconazole (Nizoral)

Labetolol (Trandate)

Lithium

Lorazepam

Medroxyprogesterone acetate (Provera, Depo-Provera)

Megestrol (Megace)

Methadone

Methyldopa (Aldomet)

Metoclopramide (Maxolon)

Metoprolol (Lopressor)

Nadolol (Corgard)

Nizatidine

Nortriptyline (Allegron)

Oxazepam

Phenelzine (Nardil)

Phenytoin (Epanutin)

Pindolol (Viskaldix)

Prochlorperazine (Stemetil)

Progesterone (Cyclogest, Crinone, Gestone, Utrogestan, Lubion)

Propranolol (Inderal)

Ranitidine (Zantac)

Risperidone (Risperdal)

Spironolactone (Aldactone)

Temazepam

Timolol (Prestim)

Tranylcypromine (Parnate)

Trimipramine (Surmontil)

From The Multi-Orgasmic Woman *(Chia and Abrams, Harper Collins, 2005)*

Orgasm-Inhibiting Recreational Drugs

Alcohol (more than one 350ml beer, 150ml glass of wine, shot [45ml] spirits)

Tobacco (cigarettes, vapes, chewing tobacco)

Speed, cocaine, crack (uppers)

Heroin and all prescription narcotics (downers)

Ecstacy

APPENDIX B

Professional Resources

For most of these services, your first port of call will probably be your GP, who may be able to prescribe certain treatments on the NHS, or recommend a practitioner to you.

Finding an Integrative or Holistic Practitioner

- British College of Integrative Medicine (BCIM): www.integrativemedicine.uk.com
- Royal London Hospital for Integrated Medicine: www.uclh.nhs.uk
- Integrative Health Education: www.integrativehealth.co.uk
- Complementary and Natural Healthcare Council: www.cnhc.org.uk

NATUROPATHIC PHYSICIANS
- College of Naturopathic Medicine UK: www.naturopathy-uk.com

Finding an Acupuncture and Traditional Chinese Medicine Practitioner

- British Acupuncture Council: www.acupuncture.org.uk
- Association of Traditional Chinese Medicine & Acupuncture UK (ATCM): www.atcm.co.uk

Finding a Chiropractor

- British Chiropractic Association: www.chiropractic-uk.co.uk

- www.nhs.uk/Conditions/chiropractic
- International Chiropractors Association (ICA): www.icachiro.wildapricot.org/Find-a-Doctor
- World Federation of Chiropractic: www.wfc.org

Finding a Therapist

GENERAL THERAPISTS
- Royal College of Psychiatrists: www.rcpsych.ac.uk/
- British Psychological Society: www.bps.org.uk
- British Association for Counselling & Psychotherapy (BACP): www.bacp.co.uk
- Relate: www.relate.org.uk
- www.counselling-directory.org.uk

THERAPISTS SPECIALIZING IN TRAUMA RECOVERY AND WORKING WITH BODY SENSATION AND INTELLIGENCE
- Somatic Trauma Therapy London: www.somatictraumatherapy-london.com
- Somatic Experiencing Association UK: www.seauk.org.uk
- Sensorimotor Psychotherapy UK: www.sensorimotorpsychotherapy.org/referral/prUK
- Oxford Development Centre: www.oxforddevelopmentcentre.co.uk
- EMDR (Eye Movement Desensitization and Reprocessing): www.edmr.org.uk
- www.cognitivetherapy
- Mindfulness Based Cognitive Therapy (MBCT): www.mbct.cu.uk
- Help for Heroes: www.helpforheroes.org.uk
- Post Traumatic Stress Disorder: www.ptsd.org.uk

THERAPISTS SPECIALIZING IN SEXUALITY
- College of Sexual and Relationship Therapists (COSRT): www.cosrt.org.uk/
- Institute of Psychosexual Medicine: www.ipm.org.uk/
- Relate – The Relationship People: www.relate.org.uk
- www.psychosexualtherapy.org.uk

COUPLES' THERAPISTS

- The Gottman Institute: www.gottman.com/couples/private-therapy/
- The Relationship Centre: www.therelationshipcentre.org.uk
- London Emotionally Focussed Therapy Institute: www.londonefftinstitute.co.uk
- Relate – The Relationship People: www.relate.org.uk
- www.itsgoodtotalk.org.uk

For a Current Crisis

- Samaritans: www.samaritans.co.uk
- PAPYRUS – UK charity dedicated to the prevention of young suicide: www.papyrus-org.uk
- Support Line – confidential emotional support: www.supportline.org.uk
- www.nationaldomesticviolencehelpline.org.uk

Mindfulness-Based Stress Reduction (MBSR)

- Mindfulness Based Cognitive Therapy (MBCT): www.mbct.cu.uk
- The Mindfulness Centre of Excellence London UK: www.mindfulnesscentreofexcellence.com
- www.bemindful.co.uk
- Guided Mindfulness Meditations with founder John Kabat-Zinn, PhD: www.mindfulnesscds.com
- MBSR Online Course: www.soundstrue.com/store/the-mbsr-online-course-3226.html
- Search for local MBSR classes in your area!

Guided Meditation

- The Healing Mind (Dr Martin Rossman, MD): www.thehealingmind.org

Finding a Supportive Women's Group

- National Women's Register: www.nwr.org.uk

Other Books by Dr Rachel

The Man's Guide to Women: Scientifically Proven Secrets from the 'Love Lab' about What Women Really Want, by John Gottman, PhD, and Julie Schwartz Gottman, PhD, with Douglas Abrams and Rachel Carlton Abrams, MD (Rodale Books: 2016)

The Multi-Orgasmic Couple: Sexual Secrets Every Couple Should Know, by Mantak Chia, Maneewan Chia, Douglas Abrams, and Rachel Carlton Abrams, PhD (HarperOne: 2002)

The Multi-Orgasmic Woman: Sexual Secrets Every Woman Should Know, by Mantak Chia and Rachel Carlton Abrams, MD (HarperOne: 2010)

Books by Other Authors

10 Lessons to Transform Your Marriage: America's Love Experts Share Their Strategies for Strengthening Your Relationship, by John M. Gottman, PhD, Julie Schwartz Gottman, PhD, and Joan DeClaire (Harmony: 2007)

The Anatomy of a Calling: A Doctor's Journey from the Head to the Heart and a Prescription for Finding Your Life's Purpose, by Lissa Rankin, MD (Rodale Books: 2015)

And Baby Makes Three: The Six-Step Plan for Preserving Marital Intimacy and Rekindling Romance after Baby Arrives, by John M. Gottman, PhD, and Julie Schwartz Gottman, PhD (Three Rivers Press: 2007)

The Blood Sugar Solution: The UltraHealthy Programme for Losing Weight, Preventing Disease, and Feeling Great Now! by Mark Hyman, MD (Little, Brown and Company: 2012)

The Definitive Guide to Cancer, 3rd Edition: An Integrative Approach to Prevention, Treatment, and Healing, by Lise Alschuler, ND, and Karolyn A. Gazella (Celestial Arts: 2010)

Emergence of the Sensual Woman: Awakening Our Erotic Innocence, by Saida Désilets, PhD (Jade Goddess Publishing, 2006)

Finding Your Way in a Wild New World: Reclaim Your True Nature to Create the Life You Want, by Martha Beck (Free Press: 2012)

Full Body Presence: Explorations, Connections, and More to Experience Present Moment Awareness, by Suzanne Scurlock-Durana (Healing from the Core Media, 2008)

Guided Imagery for Self-Healing: An Essential Resource to Anyone Seeking Wellness, by Martin L. Rossman, MD (H. J. Kramer/New World Library: 2000)

Healing Trauma: A Pioneering Programme for Restoring the Wisdom of Your Body (with CD), by Peter A. Levine, PhD (Sounds True: 2008)

Healthy at 100: The Scientifically Proven Secrets of the World's Healthiest and Longest-Lived Peoples, by John Robbins (Ballantine Books: 2007)

The Heart Speaks: A Cardiologist Reveals the Secret Language of Healing, by Mimi Guarneri, MD, FACC (Touchstone: 2007)

The Hormone Cure: Reclaim Balance, Sleep and Sex Drive; Lose Weight; Feel Focused, Vital, and Energized Naturally with the Gottfried Protocol, by Sara Gottfried, MD (Scribner: 2014)

In an Unspoken Voice: How the Body Releases Trauma and Restores Goodness, by Peter A. Levine, PhD (North Atlantic Books: 2010)

In Defence of Food: An Eater's Manifesto, by Michael Pollan (Penguin Books: 2008)

Love and Survival: 8 Pathways to Intimacy and Health, by Dean Ornish, MD (William Morrow: 1999)

Mind Over Medicine: Scientific Proof That You Can Heal Yourself, by Lissa Rankin, MD (Hay House, Inc.: 2014)

The New Good Life: Living Better Than Ever in an Age of Less, by John Robbins (Ballantine Books: 2010)

The Seven Principles for Making Marriage Work: A Practical Guide from the Country's Foremost Relationship Expert, by John M. Gottman, PhD, and Nan Silver (Harmony: 2015)

The Spectrum: A Scientifically Proven Programme to Feel Better, Live Longer, Lose Weight, and Gain Health, by Dean Ornish, MD (Ballantine Books: 2008)

Taking Charge of Your Fertility: The Definitive Guide to Natural Birth Control, Pregnancy Achievement, and Reproductive Health (20th Anniversary Edition), by Toni Weschler (William Morrow: New York, 2015)

Ultraprevention: The 6-Week Plan That Will Make You Healthy for Life, by Mark Hyman, MD, and Mark Liponis, MD (Scribner: 2003)

Whole Body Intelligence: Get Out of Your Head and Into Your Body to Achieve Greater Wisdom, Confidence, and Success, by Steve Sisgold (Rodale Books: 2015)

The Wisdom of Menopause (Revised Edition): Creating Physical and Emotional Health During the Change, by Christiane Northrup, MD (Hay House: 2012)

Women's Bodies, Women's Wisdom (Revised Edition): Creating Physical and Emotional Health and Healing, by Christiane Northrup, MD (Bantam: 2010)

Women's Encyclopedia of Natural Medicine: Alternative Therapies and Integrative Medicine for Total Health and Wellness, by Tori Hudson, ND (McGraw-Hill Education: 2007)

Acknowledgements

To my agent, husband, playmate, idea architect and hottie, Doug Abrams, this book would not exist without you on so many levels, from conception (you are the consummate literary coach) to skilled agenting to being the kind of husband and life partner who fiercely supports my dreams and picks me up and dusts me off when I fall down. I wouldn't be the 'me' who wrote this book without your wholehearted love for my whole, sometimes messy, self.

To my unbelievably hardworking and brilliant editor, Leah Miller, thank you for your ongoing belief in this book and your careful shaping, which has made it as good as it is. Gratitude to Gail Gonzales, Jennifer Levesque, Kathleen Schmidt, Anna Cooperberg, Emily Weber Eagan, Angie Giammarino, Suzee Skwiot, and everyone else at Rodale who helped make this book a reality. Special thanks to Maria Rodale – brilliant leader of Rodale Inc., inspirational woman, mum, writer, and friend.

To my amazing doctor-writer friends who have inspired me and made me laugh out loud at what a blessed, crazy path this is: Lissa Rankin, Molly Roberts, and Sara Gottfried. Thanks for your support and feedback at all stages of the process. And to my beloved mentor, Gladys McGarey, MD, who inspires me and so many other physicians to be our best selves with our patients and to practise love as we practise medicine, as love is the true healer. Thank you for encouraging me not to give up medicine – to persist and find a practice of holistic medicine that I can love with my whole heart. And to the inspiring integrative practitioners, friends, and mentors who have paved the way for better medicine and love in the healing: Molly Roberts, Bruce Roberts, Patrick Hannaway, Wendy Warner, Scott and Suze Shannon, Jennifer Blair, Karen Lawson, Mimi Guarneri, John Weeks, Bill Manahan, Alan Gaby, Daniel Friedland, Bill Meeker, David Riley, Dean Ornish, Mark

Hyman, Tabatha Parker, and Lee Lipsenthal, may your memory be for a blessing.

Thanks to my amazing friends and sisters in the creative and online space for your tutoring of this online Neanderthal – your real friendship means the world to me: Sage Lavine, Saida Desilēts, and Sol Sebastian. And thanks to my partner in Woven (wovenweb.com), Monika Szamko, for your beautiful example of how we can be mums, change-makers, world dreamers, and intrepid world travellers. Thank you for who you are and for what you do for women everywhere. And to my inspiring sister friends, Nina Simons, Rachel Bagby, Peggy Callahan, Debora Bubb, Heather Kuiper, Mpho Tutu, Alanis Morissette, and Pam Omidyar – whose pivotal work is creating a world that we can all live in in peace. And to Father Desmond Tutu – my inspiration and spiritual mentor.

For my sister (for real), Lisa Carlton, blessed angel of my life; I can't believe we get to be sisters, friends, partners in Woven, workshop leaders, and share families and Thanksgiving dinner. I love you from here to eternity and plan to be in a rocking chair with you in about 40 years. Thanks for saving my young self.

For my women's group, which holds my soul together when it's falling apart, I couldn't do it without you: Victoria, Marie, Carey, Cat, and Valerie Joi – love you, We-ho's. And to Patty Hinz, gifted reader, doctor, photographer, and friend. Thank you for making my life more beautiful in every way.

For the goddesses and gifted healers that I am privileged to work with, you continue to blur the lines between work, fun, community, and friendship – and I love it, and all of you. Our mutual patients are so lucky to live in the sea of love you offer: Marie Royer, Adrianna Gonzalez, Aimée Gould Shunney, Lena Axelsson, Nina Kolbe, and Glynis Taormina. You inspire me daily.

For the community of patients that I have been privileged to companion on their own journeys. You surprise and inspire me on a daily basis, with your bravery, persistence, sweet vulnerability, and heartfulness. You are my best teachers.

For my beach volleyball crew in Santa Cruz – you know who you are – you keep me sane and are sometimes kind enough to let me feel like a badass. Thank you. You are my Prozac.

For my family: Mum and Dad, Irene and Don Carlton – thank you for always believing in me and telling me I could do anything I wanted, and doing everything in your power to make it so. For my brother, Jeff, sisters Lisa and Rita, nephews Grant, Andrew, Elijah, and Jordan. And for my other family, Dick and Patricia Abrams, Karen, Matt, and Halleli and Joe and Jen and Jonas. I've got your backs and I know you've got mine, and that means the world to me.

My gratitude knows no bounds for each of my blessed children: Jesse, Kayla, and Eliana. Jesse, you teach me patience, the soul gift of music, and the importance of spontaneous joy, as well as loving with your whole heart. Kayla, you teach me perseverance, what is possible when you give your all, and the importance of making a difference in the world. Eliana, you teach me to be myself, without concern for what others think, to combine science and style with sass, and to find beauty and comfort in nature and a finely crafted brunch. Each one of you has a big, beautiful, loving heart, and I am lucky to be connected to you in this lifetime.

And my forever gratitude to the Great Spirit/Mother Earth/God/Adonai Eloheinu/Goddess – the oneness that unites us all, with love and gratitude.

Endnotes

Chapter 1

1 J. Barth, L. Bermetz, E. Heim, S. Trelle, and T. Tonia. 'The Current Prevalence of Child Sexual Abuse Worldwide: A Systematic Review and Meta-Analysis.' *International Journal of Public Health* 58 (3) (2013): 469–83. doi: 10.1007/s00038-012-0426-1. Epub 2012 Nov 21.

2 This is brilliantly explored in *Mind Over Matter: Scientific Proof That You Can Heal Yourself,* by Lissa Rankin, *if* you want to read further about our bodies' *amazing* ability to heal themselves.

3 Rollin McCraty, Mike Atkinson, and Raymond Trevor Bradley. 'Electrophysiological Evidence of Intuition: Part 1. The Surprising Role of the Heart.' *Journal of Alternative and Complementary Medicine* 10 (1) (2004): 133–43.

Chapter 2

1 Toni Weschler. *Taking Charge of Your Fertility: The Definitive Guide to Natural Birth Control, Pregnancy Achievement, and Reproductive Health* (20th anniv. ed.) (William Morrow: New York, 2015).

2 John G. West, Nimmi S. Kapoor, Shu-Yuan Liao, June W. Chen, Lisa Bailey, and Robert A. Nagourney. 'Case Report: Multifocal Breast Cancer in Young Women with Prolonged Contact between Their Breasts and Their Cellular Phones.' *Case Reports in Medicine*, 2013.

3 Martha Beck. *Finding Your Way in a Wild New World: Reclaim Your True Nature to Create the Life You Want* (Free Press: New York City, 2012), xxiv.

4 Steve Sisgold. *Whole Body Intelligence: Get Out of Your Head and Into Your Body to Achieve Greater Wisdom, Confidence, and Success* (Rodale Books: New York, 2015).

Chapter 3

1 R. L. Beckstrand and J. S. Pickens. 'Beneficial Effects of Magnesium Supplementation.' *Journal of Evidence-Based Complementary and Alternative Medicine* 16 (3) (2011): 181–89.

2 I. M. Cox, M. J. Campbell, and D. Dowson. 'Red Blood Cell Magnesium and Chronic Fatigue Syndrome.' *Lancet* 337 (8744) (1991 Mar 30): 757–60.

3 G. Moorkens, Y. Manuel, et al. 'Magnesium Deficit in a Sample of the Belgian Population Presenting with Chronic Fatigue.' *Magnesium Research* 10 (1997): 329–37.

4 Seee www.nhs.uk/condition/chronic-fatigue-syndrome/pages/introduction. aspx for full definition.

Chapter 4

1 N. Torrance, B. H. Smith, M. I. Bennett, and A. J. Lee. 'The Epidemiology of Chronic Pain of Predominantly Neuropathic Origin. Results from a General Population Survey.' *Journal of Pain* 7 (4) (2006): 281–89.

2 *Global Burden of Disease Report* (2010).

3 A. M. Elliott, B. H. Smith, K. I. Penny, W. C. Smith, and W. A. Chambers. 'The Epidemiology of Chronic Pain in the Community.' *Lancet* 354 (1999): 1248–252.

4 P. Posadzki, et al. 'Is Yoga Effective for Pain? A Systematic Review of Randomized Clinical Trials.' *Complementary Therapies in Medicine* 19 (5) (2011 Oct.): 281–87.

5 James A. Duke. 'The Garden Pharmacy: Turmeric, the Queen of COX-2 Inhibitors.' *Alternative and Complementary Therapies* 13(5) (November 2007): 229–34.

6 Alexandra Sifferlin. 'The Problem with Treating Pain in America.' *Time* (January 12, 2015).

Chapter 5

1 Edward O. Laumann, John H. Gagnon, Robert T. Michael, and Stuart Michaels. 'National Health and Social Life Survey.' The National Opinion Research Center at the University of Chicago, 1992.

2 C. Gingell, D. Glasser, E. Laumann, E. Moreira, A. Nicolosi, and T. Wang. 'Sexual Problems among Women and Men Aged 40–80 Y: Prevalence and Correlates Identified in the Global Study of Sexual Attitudes and Behaviours.' *International Journal of Impotence Research* 17 (1) (2005): 39–57.

3 R. Nappi, S. Detaddei, F. Ferdeghini, B. Brundu, A. Sommacal, and F. Polatti. 'Role of Testosterone in Feminine Sexuality.' *Journal of Endocrinological Investigation* 26, suppl. 3 (2003): 97–101.

4 S. R. Davis and J. Tran. 'Testosterone Influences Libido and Well-Being in Women.' *Trends in Endocrinology and Metabolism* 12 (1) (2001): 33–7.

Chapter 6

1 E. McGrath, G. P. Keita, B. R. Strickland, and N. F. Russo. 'Women and Depression: Risk Factors and Treatment Issues.' American Psychological Association. Washington, DC: 1990.

2 J. C. Fournier, et al. 'Antidepressant Drug Effects and Depression Severity: A Patient-Level Meta-Analysis.' *Journal of the American Medical Association* 303 (1) (2010): 47–53.

3 I. Kirsch, et al. 'Initial Severity and Antidepressant Benefits: A Meta-Analysis of Data Submitted for the Food and Drug Administration.' *PLOS Medicine* 5 (2) (2008): 45.

4 J. Rush, et al. 'Acute and Longer-Term Outcomes in Depressed Outpatients Requiring One or Several Treatment Steps: A STAR*D Report.' *American Journal of Psychiatry* 163 (2006): 1905–1917.

5 Scott Shannon. 'The Ecology of Mental Health' from presentation at the American Board of Integrative Medicine conference (11/6/2013).

6 L. M. Jaremka, R. R. Andridge, C. P. Fagundes, C. M. Alfano, S. P. Povoski, A. M. Lipari, D. M. Agnese, M. W. Arnold, W. B. Farrar, L. D. Yee, W. E. Carson III, T. Bekaii-Saab, E. W. Martin Jr., C. R. Schmidt, and J. K. Kiecolt-Glaser. 'Pain, Depression, and Fatigue: Loneliness as a Longitudinal Risk Factor.' *Health Psychology* 33 (9) (2014 Sept.): 948–57. doi: 10.1037/a0034012. Epub 2013 Aug 19.

7 Rollin McCraty, et al. 'The Impact of a New Emotional Self-Management Programme on Stress, Emotions, Heart Rate Variability, DHEA, and Cortisol.' *Integrative Physiological and Behavioural Science* 33, no. 2 (April-June 1998): 151–70.

8 Rollin McCraty. 'The Effects of Emotions on Short-Term Power Spectrum Analysis of Heart Rate Variability.' *American Journal of Cardiology* 76, no. 14 (November 15, 1995): 1089–93.

9 D. Babyak, et al. 'Exercise Treatment for Major Depression: Maintenance of Therapeutic Benefit at 10 Months.' *Psychosomatic Medicine* 62 (2000): 633–38.

10 Mahmood Bakhtiyari, et al. 'Anxiety as a Consequence of Modern Dietary Pattern in Adults in Tehran – Iran.' *Eating Behaviours* 4, issue 2 (April 2013): 107–12.

11 J. L. Hibbeln. 'Fish Consumption and Major Depression.' *Lancet* 351 (1998): 1213.

12 Raymond W. Lam, et al. 'Efficacy of Bright Light Treatment, Fluoxetine, and the Combination in Patients with Non-Seasonal Major Depressive Disorder.' *JAMA Psychiatry* 73 (1) (2016): 56–63.

13 K. Shaw, J. Turner, and C. Del Mar. 'Are Tryptophan and 5-Hydroxytryptophan Effective Treatments for Depression? A Meta-

Analysis.' *Australian and New Zealand Journal of Psychiatry* 36 (4) (2002 Aug.): 488–91.

14 S. J. Lewis. 'Folic Acid Supplementation during Pregnancy May Protect against Depression 21 Months after Pregnancy, an Effect Modified by MTHFR C677T Genotype.' *European Journal of Clinical Nutrition* 66 (1) (2011): 97–103.

15 Arnold Mech and Andrew Farah, 'Correlation of Clinical Response with Homocysteine Reduction During Therapy with Reduced B Vitamins in Patients with MDD Who Are Positive for MTHFR C677T or A1298C Polymorphism: A Randomized, Double-Blind, Placebo-Controlled Study.' *Journal of Clinical Psychiatry* 77 (5) (2016): 668–71.

16 A. Palatnik, K. Frolov, M. Fux, J. Benjamin. 'Double-Blind, Controlled, Crossover Trial of Inositol versus Fluvoxamine for the Treatment of Panic Disorder.' *Journal of Clinical Psychopharmacology* (3) (2001 June 21): 335–39.

17 I. K. Lyoo, et al. 'A Randomized, Double-Blind Placebo-Controlled Trial of Oral Creatine Monohydrate Augmentation for Enhanced Response to a Selective Serotonin Reuptake Inhibitor in Women with Major Depressive Disorder.' *American Journal of Psychiatry* 169 (9) (2012): 937–45.

18 K. Linde, M. M. Berner, and L. Kriston. 'St. John's Wort for Major Depression.' *Cochrane Database of Systematic Reviews* 4 (2008 October).

19 C. F. Haskell, et al. 'The Effects of L-Theanine, Caffeine and Their Combination on Cognition and Mood.' *Biological Psychiatry* 77 (2) (2008): 113–22.

20 R. Leo, et al. 'A Systematic Review of Randomized Controlled Trials of Acupuncture in the Treatment of Depression.' *Journal of Affective Disorders* 97 (2007): 13–22.

21 K. Pilkington, G. Kirkwood, H. Rampes, M. Cummings, and J. Richardson. 'Acupuncture for Anxiety and Anxiety Disorders – A Systematic Literature Review.' *Acupunctural Medicine* 25 (1-2) (2007 June): 1–10.

Chapter 7

1 J. M. Smyth. 'Effects of Writing about Stressful Experiences on Symptom Reduction in Patients with Asthma or Rheumatoid Arthritis: A Randomized Trial.' *Journal of the American Medical Association* 281 (14) (1999 Apr 14): 1304–9.

Chapter 8

1 Eric Schlosser. *Fast Food Nation: The Dark Side of the All-American Meal* (Mariner Press: New York, 2012).

2 CDC, Division of Nutrition, Physical Activity, and Obesity, National Center for Chronic Disease Prevention and Health Promotion, September 21, 2015.

3 Environmental Working Group, 2005.

4 L. Oates, et al. 'Reduction in Urinary Organophosphate Pesticide Metabolites in Adults after a Week-Long Organic Diet.' *Environmental Research* 132 (2014): 105–11.

5 Environmental Working Group, ewg.org, 2016.

6 Michael Pollan. *In Defense of Food: An Eater's Manifesto* (Penguin Books: New York, 2008).

7 I. Hu Yang, et al. 'Coconut Oil: Non-alternative Drug Treatment Against Alzheimer's Disease.' *Nutricion Hospitalaria* (Madrid) 32 (6) (2015 Dec 1): 2822–27.

8 W. M. Fernando, et al. 'The Role of Dietary Coconut for the Prevention and Treatment of Alzheimer's Disease: Potential Mechanisms of Action.' *British Journal of Nutrition* 114 (1) (2015 July 14): 1–14.

Chapter 9

1 S. W. Lockley, G. C. Brainard, and C. A. Czeisler. 'High Sensitivity of the Human Circadian Melatonin Rhythm to Resetting by Short Wavelength Light.' *Journal of Clinical Endocrinology and Metabolism* 88 (9) (2003): 4502–5.

2 M. Hysing, S. Pallesen, K. M. Stormark, R. Jakobsen, A. J. Lundervold, and B. Sivertsen. 'Sleep and Use of Electronic Devices in Adolescence: Results from a Large Population-Based Study.' *BMJ Open* 5 (1) (2015): e006748.

3 Jacob Schor. 'Life through Orange-Coloured Glasses: Blue-Blocking Lenses May Alleviate Sleep Disruption in Teens.' *Natural Medicine Journal* 7, issue 9 (September 2015).

4 B. Abbasi, et al. 'The Effect of Magnesium Supplementation on Primary Insomnia in Elderly: A Double-Blind Placebo-Controlled Clinical Trial.' *Journal of Research in Medical Science* 17 (12) (2012 Dec): 1161–69.

5 J. F. Duffy, D. J. Dijk, E. B. Klerman, and C. A. Czeisler. 'Later Endogenous Circadian Temperature Nadir Relative to an Earlier Wake Time in Older People.' *American Journal of Physiology* 275 (5 Pt 2) (November 1998): R1478–R1487.

6 D. J. Dijk, J. F. Duffy, and C. A. Czeisler. 'Contribution of Circadian Physiology and Sleep Homeostasis to Age-Related Changes in Human Sleep.' *Chronobiology International* 17 (3) (2000 May): 285–311.

Chapter 10

1 G. D. Lewis, et al. 'Metabolic Signatures of Exercise in Human Plasma.' *Science Translational Medicine* 2 (33) (2010, May 26): 33ra37.

2 Gregory N. Bratman, et al. 'The Benefits of Nature Experience: Improved Affect and Cognition.' *Landscape and Urban Planning* 138 (June 2015): 41–50.

3 N. Sydó, et al. 'Relationship between Exercise Heart Rate and Age in Men vs. Women.' *Mayo Clinic Proceedings* 89 (12) (2014 Dec): 1664–72. doi:10.1016/j.mayocp.2014.08.018. Epub 2014 Oct 29.

4 L. A. Tucker, J. E. Strong, J. D. LeCheminant, B. W. Bailey. 'Effect of Two Jumping Programmes on Hip Bone Mineral Density in Premenopausal Women: A Randomized Controlled Trial.' *American Journal of Health Promotion.* 29 (3) (2015 Jan-Feb): 158-64.

5 S. J. Allison, K. E. S. Poole, G. M. Treece, et al. 'The Influence of High-Impact Exercise on Cortical and Trabecular Bone Mineral Content and 3D Distribution Across the Proximal Femur in Older Men: A Randomized Controlled Unilateral Intervention.' *Journal of Bone and Mineral Research.* Published online August 17, 2015.

6 K. Gebel, et al. 'Effect of Moderate to Vigorous Physical Activity on All-Cause Mortality in Middle-Aged and Older Australians.' *Journal of the American Medical Association Internal Medicine* 175 (6) (2015 June): 970–77.

7 T. Sijie, Y. Hainai, Y. Fengying, and W. Jianxiong. 'High-Intensity Interval Exercise Training in Overweight Young Women.' *Journal of Sports Medicine and Physical Fitness* 52 (3) (2012): 255–62.

8 L. Gliemann, et al. '10-20-30 Training Increases Performance and Lowers Blood Pressure and VEGF in Runners.' *Scandinavian Journal of Medicine and Science in Sports* 25 (5) (Oct. 2015): e479–89. doi: 10.1111/sms.12356. Epub 2014 Dec 1.

Chapter 11

1 Rollin McCraty, Mike Atkinson, and Raymond Trevor Bradley, 'Electro-physiological Evidence of Intuition: The Surprising Role of the Heart,' *Journal of Alternative and Complementary Medicine* 10(1) (2004): 133–43.

2 J. S. House, K. R. Landis, and D. Umberson. 'Social Relationships and Health.' *Science* 241 (1988): 540–45.

3 Dean Ornish. *Love and Survival: 8 Pathways to Intimacy and Health* (William Morrow: New York, 1999): 13.

4 Debra Umberson and Jennifer Karas Montez. 'Social Relationships and Health: A Flashpoint for Health Policy.' *Journal of Health and Social Behaviour* 51, 1 suppl. (November 2010): S54–S66.

5 S. Levine, D. M. Lysons, and A. F. Schatzberg. 'Psychobiological Consequences of Social Relationships.' *Annals of the New York Academy of Sciences* 807 (1997): 210–18.

6 A. Rosengren, et al. 'Stressful Life Events, Social Support, and Mortality in Men Born in 1933.' *British Medical Journal* 307 (6912) (Oct. 19, 1993): 1102–5.

7 S. Cohen. 'Social Supports and Physical Health.' In: A.L. Greene, M. Cummings, K.H. Karraker, eds. *Life-Span Developmental Psychology: Perspectives on Stress and Coping* (Hillsdale, NJ: Erlbaum Associates, 1991).

8 S. Cohen, et al. 'Social Ties and Susceptibility to the Common Cold,' *Journal of the American Medical Association* 277 (1997): 1940–44.

Chapter 12

1 Marge Piercy. *Circles on the Water.* (Alfred A. Knopf: New York) 1982.

2 D. Oman, C. Thoresen, and K. McMahon, 'Volunteerism and Mortality Among the Community Dwelling Elderly.' *Journal of Health Psychology* 4(3) (May 1999): 301–16.

3 M. Moreno, F. Furtner, and F. Rivara, 'Adolescent Volunteering.' *JAMA Pediatrics* 167(4) (2013): 400.

4 T. N. Alim, A. Feder, et al. 'Trauma, Resilience, and Recovery in a High-Risk African-American Population,' *American Journal of Psychiatry* 165(12) (Dec. 2008): 1566–75.

5 Social Capital Community Benchmark Survey. The Saguaro Seminar. Harvard Kennedy School, 2006.

6 Allan Luks. 'Doing Good: Helper's High.' *Psychology Today* 22, no. 10 (1988): 34–42.

7 James Baraz and Shoshana Alexander. 'The Helper's High.' *Greater Good: The Science of a Meaningful Life* (February 1, 2010).

8 P. A. Boyle, et al. 'Effect of a Purpose in Life on Risk of Incident Alzheimer Disease and Mild Cognitive Impairment in Community-Dwelling Older Persons.' *Archives of General Psychiatry* 67 (3) (March 2010): 304–10. doi: 10.1001/archgenpsychiatry.2009.208.

9 Y. Sugihara, H. Sugisawa, H. Shibata, and K. Harada, 'Productive Roles, Gender, and Depressive Symptoms: Evidence from a National Longitudinal Study of Late-Middle-Aged Japanese.' *Journal of Gerontology* 6303(4) (2008): 227–34.

10 Y. Li, L. Xu, I. Chi, and P. Guo. 'Participation in Productive Activities and Health Outcomes among Older Adults in Urban China.' *The Gerontologist* 54(5): 784–96.

11 John Robbins. *Healthy at 100: The Scientifically Proven Secrets of the World's Healthiest and Longest-Lived Peoples (*New York: Ballantine Books, 2006).

12 Mary Oliver. 'The Summer Day' from *New and Selected Poems* (Boston: Beacon Press, 1992).

Appendix A

1 Jan L. Shifren and Margery L. S. Gass. 'The North American Menopause Society Recommendations for Clinical Care of Midlife Women,' 2016, NAMS blog, menopause.org/publications/clinical-care-recommendations.

Index

Boldface page references indicate illustrations.
Underscored references indicate boxed text.

depression, therapy for (*cont.*)
exercise 231
5-hydroxy tryptophan (5-HTP) 109
guided meditation 105
herbs 111–13, 221
hormones 113–14
innovative approaches 102
light therapy 108, 108
meditation and prayer 82
S-adenosyl methionine (SAM-e)
111
spiritual practice 104–5
support 103–4
therapists 103–4
vitamin D 109
detoxification 219–20
DHA 56, 78, 107, 128, 146, 221
diet 137–52
anti-inflammatory 215, 216
Bodywise 28-Day Plan 207–3
elimination 215–16, 218, 222–3
low-allergen 215–19, 215–19
nutritional supplements 220–1
digestive enzymes 56
diphenhydramine 165
discernment 9–11
in body quotient (BQ) quiz 14–15
BodyWise Movement exercise 42
finding 36
honing with
mindfulness/wordlessness 40–1
movement 41–2, 42
in practice 36–7
sense of purpose 196–9
setting the stage for process 40–3
through movement 41–2, 42
when is a headache just a headache
38–40
which voices to listen to 37–8
dopamine 112, 115, 140, 193
drinks 207, 214, 214
drugs. *See also* medications
diversity in the effect of xviii
libido decreasing 243
orgasm-inhibiting 242, 243
dust mites 131, 235, 238

E

earplugs 159–60, 226
eating, bodywise 141
eating plan, basic BodyWise 206–7

eczema 33–5, 40, 124, 126
eggs 129, 206, 214, 219
electrical fields 159
electrical frequencies, effect of 26–7
electronic activity tracker 19, 20, 26–8
elimination diet 215–16, 218, 222–3
emotional intelligence 8
emotions:
body posture and 41
causes of stress 51
connection to others 182
sensations related to experiences 33
endorphins 184
EPA 78, 107, 128, 146, 221
Epstein-Barr virus 61, 61
ergonomics 74, **75**
escitalopram 111
estradiol 81, 91, 95, 117, 164
estriol 91
evening primrose oil 93, 123, 126
exercise(s) 167–77
aerobic 170–2, 171, 228–9, 231
Belly Breathing 21
benefits of 167–70, 171, 173
chronic pain treatment 76–7
depression and anxiety 106
libido increase 94
sleep improvement 155
stress relief 53, 128
Body Awareness 30–1
Body Feelings 34
BodyWise Movement 42
in Bodywise 28-Day Plan 228–31
designing week plan 230
finding your perfect movement
176–7
flexibility and balance 174, 229
goals 229–30
high-intensity interval training (HIIT)
175–6, 229
intensity 175–6
Quality of Sensation 32
Shifting Pain 84
strength-building 172–4, 173, 229
Tuning In to You 'Yes' and 'No,' 9

F

fantasy 94
fatigue 47–69
chronic fatigue syndrome 65, 67,
67–8

heart disease (*cont.*)
  healthy fats 146
  social connection 192
  increase risk with depression 101
HeartMath 105–6, 178
heart rate, maximum 171, <u>172</u>
heart wisdom 178–9, 189
heavy metals 63–4
herbs:
  for adrenal recovery 53–4
  for heavy/irregular periods 57–8
  immune-enhancing 61
  for inflammation 78, <u>79</u>
  for mood support 99–100, 111–13, 221
  for sleep 161–2
high-efficiency particulate air (HEPA) filter 131, 238, 239
high-fructose corn syrup 151, <u>209</u>
high-intensity interval training (HIIT) 175–6, 229–30
hip circumference, measuring 234–5, <u>234</u>
homeostasis 51
hops gel 91
hormone-replacement therapy 113, 241–2
hormones. *See also* specific hormones
  bio-identical 57, 91, 113, 163, 241
  influence on
    depression and anxiety 113–14
    libido 92–3
    migraine headaches 81
  in menstrual cycle 24–6, 81
  sleep disruption from 163–4
  testing 81
hot flushes xvii, 93, 113, 153, 158, 163–4, 226, 241, 242
household toxin exposure <u>66</u>
humidity, low for avoiding allergens 238
hunger signals 137, <u>138</u>, 139
hydrocodone 79
hyperthyroidism 60
hypothyroidism 60, <u>68–9</u>, 93, 130

I

infections <u>61</u>, 61–2, <u>69</u>
inflammation 55
  anti-inflammatory compounds 78–80, <u>79</u>, 128

anti-inflammatory food 77–8, 107, 123, 128, 144, 146, 215, <u>216</u>
blood tests for systemic 81, <u>83</u>
causes 77–8
inflammatory food 77–8, 107
reducing for
  allergy and autoimmune conditions 128
  chronic pain relief 77–80
  systemic 77
inositol 110–11, <u>115</u>
insomnia 153–4, 159–60, 162–4, <u>166</u>
integrative medicine:
  author's practice of xi–xiii, 26
  finding a doctor 245
  inflammation reduction 77
  wired-and-tired problem 98
intestinal disorders 56
intuition 8, 72, 123, 138, 178–9
iron 56–8, <u>68</u>
isoflavones 164

K

karsai nei tsang 76
kava 102, 162

L

lavender oil 99–100, 112, <u>115</u>, 160, 162
lemon balm 160
lentils 144
libido 85–96
  drugs decreasing <u>243</u>
  health workup for low <u>95</u>
  influences on 86–95
    exercise 231
    hormonal and medical 92–3
    painful sex 90–2
    relationships 95
    social and cultural 87–8
    stress and busyness 93–4
    trauma and bad sex 88–90
  'libido reclamation' story 87
  prevalence of low sexual desire 86
  quiz 85
liquorice 54
light pollution, sleep disruption and 155–7, 225
light therapy 108, <u>108</u>
love 178–89